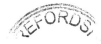

Surgery in the Surgery

Sidha Sambandan FRCGP, FRCS

Forewords by

David Haslam
Chair, Examination Board, RCGP

and

John Biggs
Regional Dean, Anglia Region

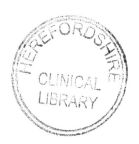

Radcliffe Medical Press

Radcliffe Medical Press Ltd
18 Marcham Road, Abingdon, Oxon OX14 1AA

British Library Cataloguing in Publication Data

A catalogue record for this book is available from the British Library.

ISBN 1 85775 284 8

Typeset by Advance Typesetting Ltd, Oxon
Printed and bound in Hong Kong

Contents

Foreword

General practice is not an easy job. Of all the medical specialities, it is the hardest to do well, and the easiest to do badly. General practitioners are busy people, with too much to do, and too little time. So why would any sensible doctor still wish to take on the challenge of minor surgery?

Much of the stress of modern day general practice stems from the difficulty in seeing a clear and obvious outcome from the doctor's work. With health promotion, blood pressure screening, diabetic management, countless new administrative duties, and many of the GP's other tasks, it is difficult to see that what you are doing is truly worthwhile – at least not until several years have passed. But with minor surgery, what you do has a clear, instant result, with the potential for very real professional fulfilment. In studies of GP stress, it has been clearly shown that the simple satisfaction gained from doing a clinical procedure well can give the doctor a real boost. It is a situation in which everyone can be a winner.

But it has to be done well. If you are like me, you may well have started a procedure and immediately regretted it. As the blood flows around the sebaceous cyst, and the wall of the cyst becomes harder to see, let alone dissect, you may find yourself asking 'why on earth did I start this? After all, I could have just referred it.'

And yet, for both patients and doctors, surgery in the surgery can be enormously rewarding. It is efficient, relatively cheap, popular and a logical way of using our skills. I am frequently embarrassed to think that the 'ChB' part of my qualifications means 'Bachelor in Surgery'. Few hard-earned university degrees can be wasted by so many graduates.

For doctors who want to extend, develop and perfect their surgical skills, Sidha Sambandan has produced this truly excellent book. Highly readable, entertaining, thought-provoking, and frequently witty and amusing, this book provides the information that general practitioners need in an accessible form. You will learn a great deal from it and should keep it close to hand for ready reference.

Books on surgery are often seen as dull, as mere collections of facts and illustrations. It's not that there is anything wrong with facts and illustrations, but few will feel that they make for a stimulating read. This book is mercifully different. Quotations (some dating back many centuries BC), epigrams, humour, reflections and references – including web sites – make this an entertaining, stimulating and extraordinarily welcome addition to the literature of general practice. I suspect mine will not be the only patients to be intensely grateful.

David Haslam
Chairman of Examination Board and
Assessment Network, RCGP
May 1999

Foreword

Medicine is changing quickly says Dr Sambandan in his Preface and the rush of new health policies and programmes in the United Kingdom makes further change inevitable. Nowhere is the potential for change greater than in general practice in England as the rapid development of primary care groups gathers pace.

But while new systems and organisational structures are put in place the essential task for the general practitioner remains the same: the best possible care of his or her patient. Dr Sambandan has promoted this quality of care for many years as general practice tutor. He has made a special contribution through his advancement of training in the principles and practice of minor surgery and his establishment of a highly successful course in minor surgery for general practitioners in Norwich.

The patient with a complaint potentially correctable by surgery will usually present first to the general practitioner for advice and management. The prospect of a long wait for an outpatient appointment and a possibly longer wait for a date for surgery will daunt many. Where the surgery is minor in degree the possibility of having a necessary procedure undertaken in the surgery by the known practitioner in known surroundings and without delay will be warmly welcomed.

It goes without saying that the practitioner must be skilled and confident in the surgical task and Dr Sambandan makes this point repeatedly. The necessary instruments and facilities must be available and the minor surgery planned and explained to the patient; there must be informed and intelligent assistance to hand; preliminary tasks must be done and removed tissue sent for histopathology. All of these necessities are well covered in the book.

Dr Sambandan has produced a robust and readily readable coverage of a topic that will challenge general practitioners both older and younger.

I expect his book to have wide appeal to general practitioners, their helpers and others called upon to undertake some of the skills described. I wish it every success.

John Biggs
Postgraduate Dean
University of Cambridge and the
Eastern Region of the National Health Service
May 1999

Preface

Reading maketh a full man;
Conference a ready man; and
Writing an exact man.

Francis Bacon

This workbook is primarily written for primary-care physicians (family practitioners or general practitioners as they are known in the United Kingdom) and practice nurses or nurse practitioners involved in minor surgical procedures in primary care. It is not intended to transmit facts, but to discuss important issues in minor surgery which need reflection. I will be more than happy to discuss any questions that may arise, when you use this workbook. The easiest way of contacting me is by e-mail on *sambandan@aol.com*. I do not profess to know all the answers though! I would also be grateful for any suggestions and comments.

You will note many quotes during your sojourn through this book. I make no apologies for them. I quote others in order to express myself better, and I share the same sentiments. Some of these quotes are thought-provoking. The origins of most of these quotes are obscure, though you will see the sources of their supposed origins. The name and fame goes to the person who disseminates the idea, and not to the person who had the original idea or uttered the aphorism.

Medicine and technology are changing so quickly that much of what is written today as fact may only be of historical interest tomorrow. Hence the importance of updating our knowledge and skills continuously, and applying it to our clinical practice. The patient is the greatest teacher, and constant reflection on our actions, review of our patient outcomes and revising our methods help in the evolution of our knowledge, skills and attitude to primary-care surgery, fulfilling the synthesis of head, hand and heart in our lifelong learning.

The main aim of this workbook is to enhance your knowledge and skills in self-directed learning, which all adults are capable of. I hope it has an impact on the five 'R's of clinical practice:

Reading (includes searching, selecting and critical appraisal of electronic information)
'R'iting (ability to write reports/assignments)
'R'ithmetic (audit and quality assessment)
'R'ticulating (communication skills)
Reflection (both in and on our clinical practice).

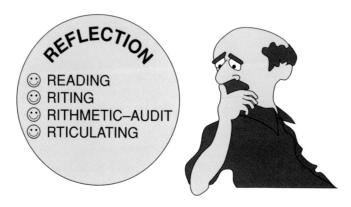

The art of learning how to learn depends on the acquisition of the above five skills.

I have here only made a nosegay of culled flowers, and have brought nothing of my own but the thread that ties them together.

Montaigne

Continuing professional development (CPD) of a practitioner is the lifelong *systematic* learning that involves the development, maintenance, improvement and broadening of his or her knowledge and skills. I have used minor surgery as an example of the way in which a practitioner could improve on the five 'R's of practice. This workbook complements the 2½-day course on minor surgery that is held twice a year in Norwich. The Norwich course is unique, since the half-day is held about 1–2 months after the first 2 days. This allows practitioners to return to their practices, observe and reflect on their current practice in their individual settings and implement any changes in the structures and processes, evaluate what they do, and document it in the form of a report or assignment. This is sent to the tutor before attending the half-day, the purpose of which is to have an objective structured clinical assessment and review (OSCAR) of minor surgery. This assessment involves 24 work-stations followed by a review of the course. This workbook, together with participation in a properly planned course, will enhance your knowledge and skills in the theory and practice of minor surgery and have an impact on your communication skills, audit and quality assurance, and ability to write reports and assignments.

I have included an overview for each chapter, which will give you an idea of the content. Some chapters will have a section on 'frequently asked questions' (FAQs); some of these are questions that arose during the courses run in Norwich, and some have been formulated to address important and relevant issues. At the end of each chapter I have included resources for references and further reading.

Sidha Sambandan
May 1999

Acknowledgements

This workbook has evolved over several years and I wish to acknowledge the support and feedback given by all my colleagues who helped me to run the course. Special mention must be made of Dr Nicholas Levell, with whom I developed the 'OSCAR' (objective structured clinical assessment and review). Others include Mr A D Patel, Dr Robin Farman, Mr Maurice Meyer, Dr Karl Gaffney, Mr Allan Bardsley, Mr Stuart Scott, Mr John Colin, Dr Clive Grattan, Dr Peter Phillips and Dr Tim Barker. Special thanks to Dr Levell and Dr Grattan for reading my drafts of chapters 6–8 and making useful suggestions. I also wish to thank Professor Rona Mackie of the Department of Dermatology, Glasgow University and Dr Clive Grattan for permission to use some of their slides in this book. Thanks are also due to Carissa Mundy for supplying the draft illustrations. Dr Bob Berrington (Regional Director in General Practice), Dr Arthur Hibble (Deputy Director), Dr Steve Lazar and Dr Christopher Hand (Assistant Directors) have supported the development of the Norwich Minor Surgery Course. Maureen Goodwin, Carol Everest and Richard Nuttall, who helped me in the organisation of the courses. A special thanks to all my friends and colleagues who have read and commented on various chapters.

Abbreviations

AMS	atypical mole syndrome
BASICS	British Association of Immediate Carers
BBV	blood-borne virus
BCC	basal cell carcinoma
BLS	basic life support
CDSC	Communicable Diseases Surveillance Centre
CHD	coronary heart disease
CME	continuing medical education
CNS	central nervous system
COSHH	Control of Substances Hazardous to Health
CPD	continuing professional development
CPR	cardiopulmonary resuscitation
CSSD	Central Sterile Supplies Department
CVS	cardiovascular system
DMN	dysplastic melanocytic naevi
DoH	Department of Health
DPU	day procedure unit
DVT	deep vein thrombosis
ELM	epiluminescence microscopy
Emla®	eutectic mixture of local anaesthetics
ENT	ear, nose and throat
EPP	exposure-prone procedure
FAQ	frequently asked questions
FB	foreign body
FP	family practitioner/physician
FULG	fulguration waveform
GA	general anaesthetic/anaesthesia
GMS	General Medical Services

GMSC	General Medical Services Committee
GP	general practitioner
HA	health authority
HAV	hepatitis A virus
HBV	hepatitis B virus
HCV	hepatitis C virus
HCW	healthcare worker
HIV	human immunodeficiency virus
HPV	human papilloma virus
IGTN	ingrowing toe-nail
IHD	ischaemic heart disease
LA	local anaesthesia/anaesthetic
MDU	Medical Defence Union
MM	malignant melanoma
MPS	Medical Protection Society
MS	minor surgery
MUA	manipulation under anaesthesia
NHS	National Health Service
NLP	neurolinguistic programming
NSAIDs	non-steroidal anti-inflammatory drugs
OSCAR	objective structured clinical assessment and review
OTC	over the counter
PBS	personal bibliographic software
PEP	post-exposure prophylaxis
PHCT	primary healthcare team
PPA	Prescription Pricing Authority
RCGP	Royal College of General Practitioners
RSI	repetitive strain injury
RSTL	relaxed skin tension line
SCC	squamous cell carcinoma
SPF	sunscreen protection factor
STD	sodium tetradecyl sulphate
UVA	ultraviolet A
VV	varicose veins
v/v	volume/volume
w/v	weight/volume
www	worldwide web

Study is WORK.
Inquiry into the value and
applicability of what is
studied is WORSHIP.
The experience of the validity and value of
the practice is WISDOM.

Sai Baba

This workbook is dedicated to Sri Sathya Sai Baba for inspiration; my wife Jo for her tolerance; my children, Natasha, Nikola and James, for their loving interruptions; and all the participants of my courses for their motivation and feedback.

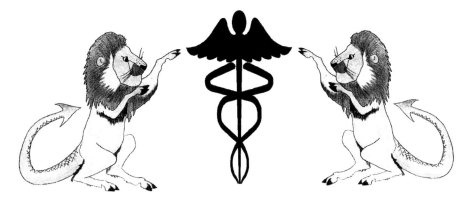

Chimera

1

Introduction

Members of the professions must build and maintain a formidable store of knowledge and skills; they must learn to absorb information through the various senses and to assess its validity, reliability and relevance. And, most importantly, they must learn to use the qualities to solve practical problems.

Heath (1990)

Minor surgery, or primary-care surgery, has now evolved into a chimeran speciality (chimera: Greek myth. A fire-breathing monster with the head of a lion, body of a goat and tail of a serpent – *see* p. xv). It demands skills acquired from different specialities, including general and plastic surgery, orthopaedics, rheumatology and dermatology. This workbook was designed to complement the 2½-day minor surgery core course that was initiated in 1995 in Norwich, and is held twice a year. Any useful course will cover the contents enumerated in Appendix B at the end of this chapter. Though it could be used on its own, as a self-study programme, it must be emphasised that the map is not the territory. *Surgery and any other technical skill can only be acquired by proper supervision and practice under supervision.* The purpose of a course is to facilitate your acquisition or maintain, update and improve your knowledge, competence and confidence in principles of the minor surgical procedures that attract a payment under the new contract of 1990. Surgery is a craft, which can only be learnt by *doing*. Aristotle said, 'For the things we have to learn before we can do them, we learn by doing them'. A course emphasises some of the issues and aspects of minor surgery, which one has to take note of while embarking on minor surgery. It is hoped that this book will be useful to gather those aspects of the knowledge base which are relevant to practice.

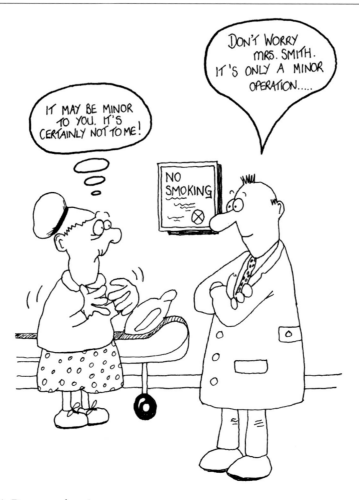

Figure 1.1 Doctor and patient.

Minor surgery is minor! However, at this moment in time, most curricula of medical schools do not ensure a demonstrable competence in minor surgical procedures in all doctors receiving the MB, BS certificate. Hence the need for a systematised introduction to the field of minor surgery. However minor the surgery may be to the surgeon, no surgery is minor to the patient.

You may already have experience of some procedures in minor surgery. The pre-course assessment questions (Appendix A) will help you decide on the areas you will need to explore further. For those already doing minor surgery, carrying out an audit on current practice and its outcome may lead to further learning needs. The General Medical Services Committee (GMSC) and Royal College of General Practitioners' (RCGP) Guidance for Minor Surgery (1997) includes guidelines on training for minor surgery not only applicable to those who wish entry into the minor surgical list of health authorities, but also to all those carrying out this work, including practitioners in private practice. This includes workshops/courses, initial clinical training in primary or secondary care under supervision by attending at least three practical sessions under approved trainers, regular updates and ensuring that standards are maintained by regular audit and educational activities. The guidelines include the content of the recommended curriculum (Appendix B) and emphasise the importance of audit at regular intervals. The Norwich minor surgery curriculum transcends a pure content-oriented curriculum and addresses the five 'R's (*see* p. x) of practice. The second half-day module is held about 6–8 weeks after the first 2-day module, allowing the participants to apply their learning and reflect on their practice, and giving time to write an assignment. The second module incorporates an objective structured clinical assessment and review (OSCAR). This helps to consolidate the learning further.

The minor surgical procedures allowed under the new contract of 1990 are given in Figure 1.2. The shaded procedures are best avoided in a primary-care setting, unless you have had prior surgical experience or training. Ganglions, especially volar surface ganglions, are best removed under good light, in an avascular field under tourniquet. Hydrocoele aspirations have a high recurrence rate, and a significant risk of infection. Exclusion of an underlying malignancy is important and, if present, there is a potential for tumour seeding. Sclerotherapy of haemorrhoids is not without problems. It requires experience and there is a distinct potential for significant haemorrhage. Those who have not had the hospital surgical experience of a Senior House Officer or higher level had best avoid them.

I will not cut for stone, even for patients in whom the disease is manifest; I will leave this operation to be performed by practitioners
Hippocrates

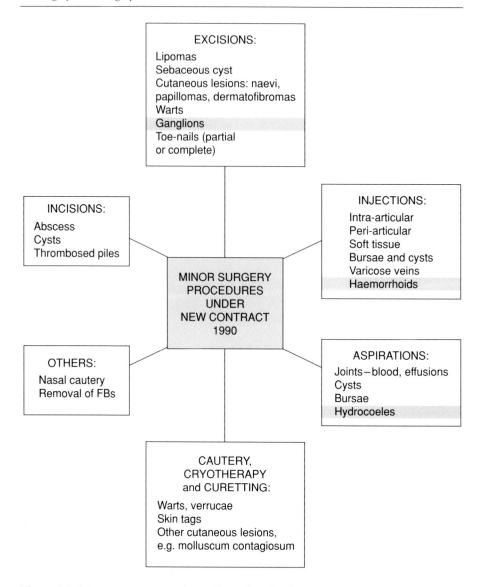

Figure 1.2 Minor surgery procedures allowed under the 1990 contract.

Self-assessment questionnaire

It will be useful for you to do a self-assessment of your current knowledge in some of the areas concerning minor surgery. The questions have been devised purely to enhance your awareness and focus your attention on some of the important issues and areas in minor surgery. Answer these as

'True' or 'False'. You could photocopy the questionnaire (Appendix A) and then write your answers on it.

Remember

It is always worth asking yourself *four questions* before attempting any surgery, anywhere on the patient:

1   *Where* is the lesion? (The anatomical *site* and the *plane*.)

2   *What* is the lesion? (The pathological *nature* of the lesion.)

3   *How* will I remove it? (Incision, access, assess, action, precautions, closure.)

4   What are my *post-operative plans*? (Advice, *follow-up of patient and lesion*.)

The golden rule:
If in doubt – REFER!

The essential skill of the surgeon is to know **WHAT** and **WHEN** to refer.

Reflections

- How will you put a patient in the recovery position? Are you skilled at it?

- Are you skilled at basic cardiopulmonary resuscitation (CPR)?

- Are you familiar with the latest protocol? When did you last practise on a manikin?

- Periodic updating of CPR skills is essential.

- Are the CPR drugs (adrenaline, hydrocortisone, chlorpheniramine and atropine) available and easily accessible in your practice?

---

*We are faced with an entirely new situation in which the **goal of education**, if we are to survive, is **the facilitation of change and learning**. The only person who is educated is the person who has **learned how to learn**; the person who has learned how to adapt and change; the person who has **realised** that no knowledge is secure, that only the **process** of seeking knowledge gives a basis of security. **Changingness,*** *a reliance on process rather than on static knowledge, is the only thing that makes any sense as a goal for education in the modern world.* [My emphasis]

Carl Rogers

Learning how to learn is about acquiring the ability to manage your time, identifying, defining, planning, implementing and reviewing what you learn. It involves skills such as lateral thinking and reflecting on what you learn, memory-enhancing techniques such as mnemonics and acronyms, creative associations and repetition. In the current ethos of accelerating change in all areas of medicine, accelerated learning and speed reading are further useful skills. Mind-mapping techniques are useful ways of generating and organising ideas, especially when writing. While most communication skills training deals with the *content* of the consultation – the *art* of consultation requires the acquisition of skills in non-verbal communication. Neurolinguistic programming (NLP) helps to enhance the visual and vocal dimensions of communication. It has been shown by Albert Mehrabian that the influence of verbal content is only 7% in communication. The non-verbal (visual) influence is 55% and the vocal influence is 38%.[1,2] This confirms the assertion that the medium *is* the message. By applying the skills of NLP, one could greatly enhance one's communication skills.

References

1   Mehrabian A. The inference of attitudes from the posture, orientation, and distance of a communication. *J Consult Psychol.* 1968; **32**: 296–308.

2   Mehrabian A. *Silent Messages.* London, Wadsworth; 1971.

Appendix A Self-assessment questionnaire

True or false?
1   The following procedures attract a minor surgery fee:
    a   injection of varicose veins
    b   removal of a foreign body from a lacerated wound of the leg
    c   vasectomy
    d   partial excision of an ingrowing toe-nail
    e   removal of a 2 mm skin tag from the neck.

2   The following statements are true:
    a   removal of two skin lesions from the same patient constitutes two separate procedures
    b   in a four-partner practice, where one partner does all the minor surgery, a claim for 12 sessions could be made per quarter by the operating partner
    c   claims cannot be carried over from one quarter to the next
    d   in order to be approved for minor surgery, an operating room of at least 17.5 m² is required
    e   a defibrillator is essential equipment in the operating room.

3   Instruments in general practice could be sterilised by:
    a   soaking in 2% glutaraldehyde for 10 minutes
    b   boiling water for 10 minutes, which will kill the spores too
    c   hot-air oven at 160°C for 1 hour
    d   autoclaving at 2.2 bar pressure, at 121°C for 15 minutes
    e   using a domestic pressure cooker at maximum pressure for 15 minutes.

4   The following statements are true, regarding local anaesthetic agents:
    a   lignocaine with 1 in 200 000 adrenaline could be used for a digital ring block
    b   the maximum safe dose of plain lignocaine is 3 mg/kg body weight
    c   the maximum adult dose is 20 ml of 1% plain lignocaine
    d   the maximum safe dose of lignocaine with adrenaline is 7 mg/kg body weight
    e   the maximum adult dose of 1% lignocaine and adrenaline is 50 ml.

5   Infections in minor surgery:
    a   could be prevented by giving prophylactic antibiotics, ideally immediately after the surgery
    b   could be prevented by always wearing surgical masks
    c   could lead to abscess formation which will need intravenous antibiotics
    d   the incidence of post-operative infections in primary care is less than in secondary care
    e   could be detected early by giving the patient appropriate post-op advice, reinforced by written instructions.

6   Bleeding during minor surgery could be controlled by:
   a   direct pressure applied for the appropriate duration
   b   applying an artery forceps, under direct vision, and tying the vessel
   c   cautery of the bleeding vessel
   d   gentle intermittent mopping with a swab
   e   packing the wound, applying compression and elevating the part for 5 minutes.

7   Keloid scarring is more likely:
   a   in incisions over the deltoid region of shoulder
   b   in sternal incisions
   c   in people of Afro-Caribbean origin
   d   in Caucasians than in Asians
   e   in posterior neck incisions.

8   The following are available on the drug tariff:
   a   Topper eight sterile multi-apertured fabric swabs 7.5 × 7.5 cm
   b   Ethilon and Prolene suture materials
   c   chromic catgut
   d   Vicryl
   e   KLING cotton conforming bandage BP – type B.

9   The following statements are true:
   a   steroid injections into the joints of poorly controlled diabetics are best avoided
   b   large lipomata in the posterior triangle of neck are best referred
   c   doctors and nurses doing minor surgery should be immunised against hepatitis A
   d   a tender, swollen knee within 48 hours after injection needs tubigrip and analgesics
   e   clinically suspicious melanomas are best referred to the hospital.

10   The following management plans are true:
   a   during nail-matrix phenolisation, 100% phenol with a 15 minute 'contact time' is adequate
   b   aspiration of a painful, swollen knee joint results in a very turbid-looking fluid; it is safe to inject steroids after aspirating completely
   c   before injecting steroids into peri- or extra-articular tissues, warn the patient about the potential cosmetic effect
   d   a firm, mobile subcutaneous lump situated 2 cm antero-inferior to the tragus, on the side of the face, can be excised under local anaesthetic quite easily

e   a patient presenting with carpal tunnel syndrome, with early thenar wasting, could be injected and monitored periodically.

11   The following statements are true regarding malignant melanomas:
   a   the prognosis depends on the 'histological thickness' of the lesion
   b   the superficial spreading melanomas are more dangerous than the nodular lesions
   c   if you make a definite clinical diagnosis, a lesion less than 1 cm is best excised with a 2 mm clear margin
   d   at least some part of the lesion is always pigmented
   e   the histology report on a melanomatous lesion comes back as 'malignant melanoma extending to the edge of the specimen'; you should follow up the patient monthly and look for clinical evidence of recurrence.

12   The following skin lesions are either pre-cancerous or cancerous:
   a   Bowen's disease
   b   histiocytomas
   c   keratoacanthoma
   d   solar keratosis
   e   rodent ulcer.

13   Curettage could be used for:
   a   seborrhoeic keratosis
   b   solitary verruca on the sole of the foot, not responding to wart paints
   c   keratoacanthoma
   d   dermatofibroma
   e   0.5 cm rodent ulcer on the face.

14   The following statements are true:
   a   always mark the skin incision pre-operatively, before excising a lesion
   b   an 'operation book' or minor surgery documentation (manual or computerised) is one of the requirements in order to be registered by the HA for minor surgery
   c   when making an elliptical incision around a cutaneous lesion, the ratio of the longitudinal axis to the transverse axis is ideally 3 : 1, with about 2 mm clearance around the edge
   d   when closing an elliptical wound, undermining the wound edges will help in suturing without tension

e   it is good practice to record your pre-operative clinical diagnosis
    of a lesion you intend to remove, and compare it with the post-
    operative histological diagnosis.

15   True or false?
     a   injecting a 'tennis elbow' could cause damage to the ulnar
         nerve
     b   Phalen's test is useful for confirming a diagnosis of carpal tunnel
         syndrome
     c   the palmaris longus is absent in some people
     d   injecting the carpal tunnel too distally could damage the palmer
         cutaneous branch of the median nerve
     e   a ganglion could be aspirated with a blue needle.

16   The following nerves could be damaged during minor surgery, due
     to the superficial distribution during their course:
     a   mandibular division of the trigeminal nerve
     b   accessory nerve
     c   axillary nerve
     d   common peroneal nerve
     e   sciatic nerve.

17   True or false?
     a   a minimum of 0.4 ml of blood is required for the transfer of
         hepatitis B virus infections in humans
     b   for the transfer of HIV, via blood, a volume of at least 1 ml is
         needed
     c   the majority of the cases of occupationally acquired HIV were
         caused by some form of sharps injury
     d   resheathing needles prior to disposal is important for the pre-
         vention of HBV transmission
     e   in the event of a sharps injury to the finger, immediate appli-
         cation of pressure is vital for prevention of HBV infection.

18   Surface temperature reductions attainable with the following
     refrigerants are:
     a   liquid nitrogen swab, $-120°C$
     b CO_2 snow, $-179°C$
     c   salt-ice, $-60°C$
     d   nitrous oxide, $-124°C$
     e   liquid nitrogen spray/probe, $-196°C$.

19 True or false?
   a   truncated neoprene cones are used in cryosurgery to concentrate the spray and limit its lateral spread
   b   otoscope earpieces are a useful alternative for limiting lateral spread of cryospray, for small lesions
   c   nail-matrix atrophy and permanent scarring are known complications of cryosurgical treatment of peri-ungual warts
   d   fibroblasts are more cryosensitive than melanocytes
   e   cryosurgery is useful for multiple viral warts of the dorsum of the hand.

20 True or false?
   a   a patient consults her GP for genital warts. It would be appropriate for her GP to treat them with cryosurgery
   b   GPs should avoid operating on feet with peripheral ischaemia
   c   early symptoms of CNS toxicity following lignocaine analgesia include: metallic taste in the mouth, tinnitus, and circumoral numbness
   d   for single-rescuer cardiopulmonary resuscitation, the UK Resuscitation Council guideline is 15 compressions for each inflation
   e   prior to excision of lumps in hairy regions, shaving of hair must be done the night before.

Answers given on page 245.

Primum non nocere
Above all do no harm

The ideal surgeon:
Must be a physician possessed of the high ideal of a Hippocrates,
The anatomical knowledge of a Vesalius,
The alertness and fearlessness of a Pare,
The intuition and curiosity of a Hunter,
The imagination of a Pasteur, and
The industry and honesty of a Lister.

Appendix B Synopsis of minor surgery courses

Guidance from the General Medical Services Committee and the Royal College of General Practitioners, in collaboration with the Royal College of Surgeons of England, Edinburgh and the British Society of Dermatological Surgery.

Administration

HA/Health board

- Rules and regulations
- Minor surgery list
  - accreditation and re-approval
- Claim procedure
  - structure of claim system
- Eligibility; numbers per month
  - money
- Payment for cases, claimable expenses

Facilities

- Premises and equipment
  - room, light, table, instruments, other equipment

Record keeping

- Clinical requirements
- HA/Health board requirements

Audit

- Requirement
- Audit cycle
  - constructive self-criticism and regular review
- Audit
  - activity, outcome, post-operative complications, malignancy, etc.

Medico-legal matters

- Duties and responsibilities, informed consent
- Written versus verbal; children and adults

Histology

- Record keeping
- Legible; contemporaneous, meticulous
- Common problems
- Avoiding pitfalls

Infection control

General

- Normal body defences
- Disinfection/sterilisation
- Staff

Sterilisation

- Methods and relative merits
  - bench-top autoclave, Central Sterile Supplies Department (CSSD), disposable instruments, hot-air sterilisers

Skin cleansing

- Health and Safety regulations
- Infection control policy
  - patients, staff
- HIV, hepatitis
  - policy for needlestick injuries, spillages, sharps disposals
- COSHH

Basic surgical techniques

Histology policy – send everything!

Planning a procedure

- Aim of procedure, explanation to patient, contingency plans

Anatomical hazards and pitfalls

- Problems
  – scarring, keloid, damage to structures, blood supply
- Danger areas – and why
  – face, neck, knee, wrist, axilla, joints, others

Designing and making an incision

- Lines of tension and creases
- Skin tension and blood supply
- Practical procedure

Instruments

- Manipulating instruments
- Recommended instruments
  – essential, desirable

Sutures

- Absorbable/non-absorbable
- Natural/synthetic

Needles

- Round-bodied and cutting

Tying knots

- Reef and granny knots, tying techniques
- Pitfalls

Suturing

- Interrupted and subcuticular

Local anaesthesia

Agents

- Types
  – lignocaine, others
- Dosage, preparations and concentrations
- Adrenaline – pros and cons

Indications and contraindications: blocks

- Local infiltration and field block
- Regional blocks (including ring blocks)

Problems

- General
  – overdose, anaphylaxis, allergy to local anaesthesia, other medical conditions
- Local
  – failure to work, danger of end arteries

Resuscitation

- Responsibility to maintain skills
- Requirements
  – facilities, equipment, staff training
- Clinical
  – recognition, action, new guidelines

Cysts, lipomas and abscesses

Epidermoid cysts

- Pathology, sites, techniques for removal
- Problems

Lipomas

- Pathology, sites, techniques for removal
- Problems

Abscesses

- Pathology, sites, problems

Miscellaneous

- Hydrocoeles
- Hormone-replacement implants
- Others

Approach to pigmented lesion

Pigmented lesions

- Benign and malignant
- Why patients present

Malignant melanoma

- Incidence
- Types
- Clinical
- Major and minor features
- Differential diagnosis
- Management
- Unexpected malignancy

Dermatological surgery

Diagnosis before treatment

- Differential diagnosis

Techniques

- Curettage, cryosurgery, electrocautery, shave excision, snipping

What to avoid

- Treatment without diagnosis, skin malignancies, inappropriate procedures, unnecessary procedures, biopsy of rashes

Varicose veins and ingrowing toe-nails

Varicose veins

- Review of surgical anatomy
- Veins suitable for injection
- Patients suitable for injection
- Indications, contraindications
  - investigations
- Technique
  - sclerosant, injection technique, bandaging
  - instruction after procedure
- Complications

Ingrowing toe-nails

- Review of surgical anatomy
- Possible treatments
  - indications, contraindications
- Local anaesthesia
- Operative techniques
- Post-operative problems

Joint and periarticular injections

Clinical conditions

- Shoulder
  - impingement syndromes, adhesive capsulitis bicipital tendonitis, others
- Elbow
  - epicondylitis
- Wrist and hand
  - de Quervain's syndrome, carpal tunnel syndrome, trigger finger
- Knee

Joints

- Examination technique
- Joints
  – shoulder, elbow, wrist and hand, knee, others

Injection

- Background
  – indications, drugs, frequency of injection, complications
- Technique
  – injection technique, asepsis, complications

The guidance also recommends that practitioners are accredited for a period of 5 years, and re-accreditation be granted so long as the practitioner has maintained adequate standards. Bear in mind that this is only a guidance on content. It is the responsibility of those who design the curriculum, not only to ensure that the content is covered, but to reflect on the methodology used and incorporate some form of evaluation to ensure that true education has been achieved, by demonstrating change.

2

Regulations and medico-legal issues

If a doctor has treated a gentleman with a bronze lancet for a severe wound and has caused him to die, or if he has opened with a bronze lancet an abscess of the eye of a gentleman and has caused the loss of the eye, the doctor's hand shall be cut off.

The code of King Hammurati (1728–1688 BC)

This chapter is written mainly in the context of primary care in the United Kingdom.

Overview

- Criteria for eligibility.
- Medico-legal aspects:
  - the golden rules
  - did you know?
  - preventing risks of litigation.

Introduction

The regulations dealing with eligibility, definition of sessions, claims and fees are dealt with in the *Red Book*, paragraphs 42.1–42.7. The criteria for selection of GPs for the minor surgery (MS) list are found in Regulation 32(3) of the *Terms Of Service*. The health authority selection criteria may vary slightly from region to region.

The procedures eligible for minor surgery fees are given in Figure 1.2. Some of the important points are:

- each GP is eligible to claim for 15 procedures (three sessions) in a quarter; five procedures constitute a session
- the procedures can be done at different times
- up to four procedures can be carried over to the next quarter
- removing two lumps from the same patient, at the same time, is counted as *two* procedures
- one partner in a practice can claim on behalf of the other partners if the latter have not done their maximum.

In December 1991 *Guidelines for Minor Surgery in General Practice* was published by the GMSC and the RCGP in collaboration with the Royal College of Surgeons of England and Edinburgh and Joint Committee on Postgraduate Training for General Practice. This guideline was updated in 1997, as was the type of training that would be required, including the 'content' of the minor surgery courses, which is given in Appendix A. Evidence of practical experience as set out by the relevant regional general practice education committee, audit, pathology and organisation, has been recommended. The importance of appropriate premises, equipment, sterilisation and safety of patients and staff was emphasised in the 1997 guidelines. Since it is important that consistent standards apply throughout the UK, they recommended that the HAs or health boards consider both *satisfactory experience* of the practitioner and *satisfactory facilities* in the practice – especially with regard to premises and equipment – to enable them to provide minor surgery services in accordance with Regulations 3B(1) and 3B(6) of the NHS General Medical Services regulations.

Criteria for eligibility to enter the MS list in Norfolk

The East Norfolk Health Authority has a *Notes of Guidance*, which lists the criteria for inclusion in the Norfolk MS list and which accompanies the application form for inclusion in the list. The criteria include competency to undertake all minor surgery procedures listed in schedule 2, paragraph 4.2 of the Statement of Fees and Allowances; a treatment room of at least 17.5 m², providing certain facilities; preparation area; and access to a list of equipment. The criteria vary from region to region.

Medico-legal aspects

Doctors bury their mistakes while lawyers hang theirs!

An excellent 14-page booklet has been issued by the Medical Defence Union (MDU) which covers all the salient medico-legal aspects of minor surgery.[1] All MDU members may acquire a free copy by contacting the MDU.

The golden rules

It requires knowledge, skills and wisdom to know when to refer.

Some of the 'golden rules' are:

1 Only carry out procedures that you are *competent and confident* in doing. What you are able to do and what you think you are able to do are not necessarily the same! It is important to remember that competence and performance do not equate to practice.[2]

2 *Select your patient carefully.* Never feel shy to refer; especially if lesions are too large or vascular, or at dangerous sites or cosmetically important areas such as the face. Consider associated illnesses, such as coronary heart disease (CHD) with dysrhythmias, diabetes, psychiatric disorders, extreme anxiety, etc. Consider current drug therapy and allergies.

Remember the five 'A's: Age, Associated illnesses, Allergies, Anticoagulants and Anxiety

- Age: especially children. Always ensure that the parent and patient understand the nature of the procedure, complications and outcomes. Avoid if child or parent is anxious.

- Associated illnesses: especially in the elderly. Consider the associated illnesses and medications the patient is having at present.

- Allergies: allergy to local anaesthetics is very rare, but asking about it is mandatory if you wish to avoid later litigation problems. Two other allergies worth asking about are whether the patient has an allergy to the skin-cleansing agents you will

continued overleaf

---

continued

use, especially iodine-containing agents, and known allergies to plaster dressings which are commonly used on the wound after an operation.

- Anticoagulants: if patients are on anticoagulants, discuss with a haematologist the timing of discontinuation and reinstitution of the drug. Aspirin and non-steroidal anti-inflammatory drugs (NSAIDs) may affect bleeding time. Some patients on aspirin tend to ooze a little more, due to the prolonged bleeding time. I do not ask patients to stop aspirin therapy for cutaneous surgery, as there is very little bleeding with these procedures and we have not experienced a greater incidence of post-operative bleeding with these patients.

- Anxious patient: AVOID operating on patients with anxiety neurosis or other mental disorders. They have unusual expectations of outcome. Procedures done for cosmetic reasons are especially vulnerable for litigation. Documented evidence about the patient being aware of the procedure, and that he or she understands the possible outcomes, is important. An appropriate consent form signed by the patient or carer is recommended.

Reflections

Avoid problem lesions,
problem sites, and
problem patients.

---

3   *Accurate documentation* of the pre-operative diagnosis, consent (written if appropriate), procedure, follow-up, complications and management are very important. An appropriate manual and/or computer record is very important (*see* Chapter 4, Appendices A and B).

4   *Communication* with the patient is essential. Always explain the nature of the problem, and the procedure you intend to do. Describe the important possible complications (e.g. scars, keloids, pigmentation, etc.) and document it. Putting the patient at ease by explaining what you are about to do – before starting the procedure – helps to reduce their anxiety and discomfort. Post-operative instructions,

especially regarding analgesia and early detection of complications such as bleeding, and action that needs to be taken, are very useful for the patient. *Written post-operative instructions* further enhance their understanding and is good practice in the current litigious culture.

5   *Organisational system*, to trace histology reports. Problems can be prevented by follow-up of all excisions at about 3–4 weeks after surgery. This will also help to pick up any incomplete excisions of unsuspected malignant lesions, which will need appropriate referral. If you keep manual records, every month a staff member (nurse or admin staff) could check the operation book to see whether all specimens sent for histology have been reported on. If the data are documented on a database, one could retrieve all excisions done in the previous month and check to see whether the histology reports have been documented.

6   *Prevention of infection*: take all the precautions necessary to reduce infection from the procedures. Surgical instruments should be properly sterilised. It is important for the staff doing minor surgery to be immunised against hepatitis B; and to take precautions to prevent hepatitis B and HIV when coming into contact with body fluids, e.g. by wearing gloves, avoiding being pricked by needles, and by appropriate disposal of used instruments and sharps. A *sharps box* to take the discarded needles and blades, and a clinical waste container, must be available close to the surgeon.

7   *Local anaesthetics*: be certain of the nature, strength and volume of anaesthetic you are about to use. *Check the contents* of the ampoule, including the *expiry date* before drawing up the local anaesthetic. It is good practice for the nurse assisting you to also check this.

8   Basic *CPR equipment and drugs* must be available and accessible. The practice nurse should ensure that the equipment is in working order, by checking periodically.

Reflections

- Will you operate on the face?

- Will you remove or refer a malignant melanoma? If so, why?

- What sort of basic CPR equipment do you have in your practice?

- What CPR drugs do you have? Are they accessible in an emergency?

- Who checks their shelf-life? How often?

continued overleaf

continued

- When will you seek help? (Uncertain diagnosis/unchartered territory/untoward event or complication/unhappy patient.) Do you have good back-up locally?

- Do you have a consent form in your practice?

- Does your consent form include a statement that the patient understands the procedure?

- Will you get written consent for all or some procedures?

- What information will you give the patient before surgery?

- What information will you give the patient after surgery?

Thou wilt also learn one necessary piece of humility, viz. Not to trust too much on thy own judgement, especially in difficult cases; but to think fit to seek advice of other Physicians or Chirurgeons.

Richard Wiseman, *Eight Surgical Treatises* (1734)

Activity

- If you do not have a consent form in your practice, devise a consent form.

- Discuss it with your partners, and revise the draft.

- Before you do the final draft, read the consent form recommended by the Medical Defence Union.[3]

Did you know?

GPs have been sued for:

- delayed diagnosis[4]/missed diagnosis of malignant lesions
- nerve damage caused by the surgeon
- infection
- not communicating an unexpected histology report of malignancy
- complications that were *not* mentioned to the patient: especially post-operative pain, haemorrhage/haematomas, sepsis, stretched/hypertrophic scars, keloids

- undertaking cosmetic procedures, especially on the face, without adequate experience or expertise.

Green[5] noted that the problems identified by the MDU relating to cosmetic surgery claims include:

1 lack of training and experience
2 poor patient selection
3 practising beyond one's competence
4 inadequate information given to the patient, i.e. informed consent
5 poor records.

> *Litigation is like a club. It's got to be used or it becomes dead-weight.*
> Victor Yannacone

The issue of *negligence* has three important components:

1 duty of care
2 breach of duty
3 the breach caused harm.

If you do not appreciate your limitations and do not know when to refer to the appropriate specialist, you become vulnerable to litigation.

Preventing the risks of litigation

The risk of litigation could be prevented by taking the following steps.

- Ask for *advice* and information from your medico-legal union before embarking on surgical procedures in primary care. This is very important if you intend to do extended procedures such as vasectomy or cosmetic procedures.
- Accurate *diagnosis*, anatomical and pathological (*clinical diagnostic skills*).
- Adequate *explanation* to the patient, *before*, *during* and *after* the surgery. (*Communication skills*, including rapport. Avoid high-risk patients [five 'A's] and high-risk areas such as the face.) It is the duty of the doctor to ensure that the patient understands the nature of the intervention, and the usual and unusual outcomes.
- Adequate *documentation* of informed consent. The issue of consent involves the mental ability of the patient to understand the information given, and consent volunteered as an autonomous individual. Do not forget to document that *informed* consent has been obtained and that the patient has been warned about possible complications (e.g.

scar/keloid). Although it is not mandatory to get written consent, it is desirable and good practice to do so, especially for removal of any lesions. It is essential to have *evidence*, in the form of documentation, that the patient has been informed and understands the possible outcomes.

- Appropriate *surgery* (*surgical skills*).
- Appropriate *risk management*. This includes:
  - reducing the risk of acquiring infection by staff, and the risk of transmitting infection to the patient
  - consent
  - adequate documentation
  - a system for the follow-up of histology
  - waste-disposal protocol
  - sharps-disposal protocol
  - storage and usage of chemicals
  - equipment usage and maintenance.
- Appropriate *post-operative instructions* about analgesia, work, complications to look for, transport back home, removal of sutures and follow-up date. A *post-operative handout* to reinforce the message is good practice.
- Appropriate *follow-up* of patient and lesion (good management systems, *organisational skills*).
- Periodic reviews, audits, significant event analysis, critical incident analysis and other *quality assurance procedures* pertaining to minor surgery are excellent ways of identifying your learning needs and facilitating the pursuit of excellence.

References

1 Dando P. *Medico-legal Aspects of Minor Surgery*. London, The Medical Defence Union Ltd; 1993.

2 Sambandan S. Competence and performance are measurable but do not equate with practice. *BMJ*. 1995; 311: 393.

3 Gilberthorpe J. Problems in general practice: Consent to treatment. In *Risk Management*, Appendix A(1), pp. 39–40. London, The Medical Defence Union Ltd; 1996.

4 *Journal of Medical and Dental Defence Union*. 1995; 11(2): 35–6.

5 Green S. Cosmetic surgery in general practice. *JMDU*. 1997; 13(1): 4–5.

Further reading

The illiterate of the future are not those who cannot read or write but those who cannot learn, unlearn and re-learn.

A. Toffler

Advisory and Risk Management Services. *Problems in General Practice Minor Surgery.* London, The Medical Defence Union Ltd; 1997.

This excellent booklet is an extension of the one below, where one organisation of medical defence has written about their experiences of analysing 26 claims over a 5-year period. It gives you an insight into the possible areas of litigation and the current trends, which show a fivefold increase in claims for vasectomy (not by definition a minor surgical procedure). A useful summary of minimising the risk of claims for the various procedures is listed.

Dando P. *Medico-legal Aspects of Minor Surgery.* London, The Medical Defence Union Ltd; 1993.

This short booklet is a must for all those embarking on minor surgery.

Gilberthorpe J. Problems in general practice: Consent to treatment. In *Risk Management*, Appendix A(1), pp. 39–40. London, The Medical Defence Union Ltd; 1996.

This consent form for medical or dental investigation, treatment or operation covers all the salient issues of consent. It is highly recommended that your consent form covers these issues.

3

Structural organisation

You cannot paint without a canvas ...
Structures precede process and outcomes

Overview

- Premises:
    - treatment room/operating room
    - lighting
    - ventilation.
- Equipment and instruments:
    - basic minor surgery equipment
    - other useful instruments
    - cautery equipment
    - electrosurgery equipment
    - radiosurgical equipment
    - cryotherapy equipment
    - sterilisers
    - resuscitation equipment and drugs
    - magnification instruments (dermatoscopy)
    - magnification loupes
    - Wood's light
    - digital photography.
- Waste disposal:
    - sharps disposal – approved container, incinerated
    - clinical waste disposal – yellow bag, incinerated

– general waste disposal – black plastic bag, sent to landfill sites for burial.

Premises

Regulations stipulate a treatment room/operating room of at least 17.5 m² (109 square feet). It is a statutory obligation to provide information, to the health authorities, on the premises and equipment to be used (Schedule 3, Part IX of GMS Regulations 1992).

The minor surgery room and equipment should ideally include:

- operating table or couch placed in a central position to be accessed from at least two sides
- operating stool (height adjustable and mobile)
- side-arm extension – especially for working on the upper limb
- sheets – disposable, or roll paper available for each patient
- adequate lighting – a movable spot lamp is very useful; good lighting is essential
- ventilation and heating
- a hand basin nearby
- washable floor; worktops and surfaces that are easy to clean
- easy access to resuscitation equipment, including drugs
- dressing trolley – don't forget to oil the wheels or castors
- sharps disposal box in close proximity
- waste disposal bin – preferably pedal-operated
- accessible telephone in close proximity
- **Steriliser**. This is the most important and expensive piece of equipment. Fortunately most practices do have a steriliser. The choice lies between a hot-air oven and an autoclave. Hot-air ovens are cheaper but the sterilising cycle is longer and the temperature higher. However, the instruments come out dry and can be stored. Autoclaves, using steam under high pressure, are more efficient, have a quicker sterilising cycle, with a lower temperature, but the instruments come out wet, and cannot therefore be stored. Neither can gauze dressing or drapes be sterilised, unless one has access to a large industrial autoclave with a pulsed vacuum cycle for drying. Instruments must be thoroughly scrubbed and cleaned before being put in a steriliser. Secretions and blood on dirty instruments become baked with heat, and sterilisation cannot then be guaranteed.

General practitioners will have access to the local hospital Central Sterile Supplies Department (CSSD) for sterilised instrument packs which can be returned for recycling. Most NHS Trusts will have a charge for lending the packs.

Equipment

Surgical instruments

Basic minor surgery pack

> *Something to hold*
> *Something to cut*
> *Something to stop bleeding*
> *Something to stitch*
> *Is all you need ...*

A list of instrument packs commonly used in general practice is given below.

BASIC MINOR SURGERY PACK – 'THE MAGNIFICENT SEVEN'

1 One scalpel handle size 3.
2 One Kilner needle holder 5¼" (13.3 cm).
3 One stitch scissors, pointed, 5" (12.7 cm).
4 One toothed dissecting forceps 5" (12.7 cm) (Gillies or Adson's).
5 Straight and curved artery forceps 5" (12.7 cm), e.g. Halsted's[1].
6 Gillies[2] skin hooks (a pair).
7 One Kilner blunt-tip curved scissors (5") (useful for tissue-plane dissection).

• One scalpel blade size 15 (size 10 and/or 11 if you prefer).
• Sterile non-absorbable suture (nylon/prolene).
• Sterile swabs.
• Sterile Tegaderm® or Opsite® to cover the wound.

(The above list is my personal favourite. You may wish to have a modified set.)

---

[1] William Halsted (1852–1922), better known for his radical mastectomy described in 1890. In 1889 he introduced rubber gloves to surgery, made by Goodyear. In 1893 he was appointed as the first Professor of Surgery at the Johns Hopkins Medical School.
[2] Sir Harrold Gillies (1882–1960). He became the first plastic surgeon at Barts.

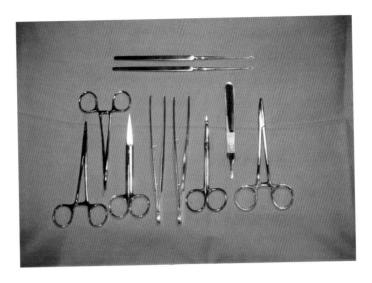

Figure 3.1 Basic minor surgery instruments.

The above seven types of instruments constitute *essential* instruments, which should be available in any practice undertaking minor surgical procedures. Items 6 and 7 are most useful for cutaneous surgery. If you are confident with your dissection ability, flat, straight or curved, pointed scissors are worthwhile acquiring. The majority of general practitioners will be doing cutaneous or subcutaneous surgery and the smaller instruments (4–6 inches) will be more appropriate. A wider range of instruments will be useful for those more experienced. It is useful to have a size 10 blade for deeper surgery, and a size 11 which is sharp and pointed. The size 11 blade is very useful for shave biopsy too. The sutures that could be prescribed are included in Chapter 9.

Other useful instruments

1 Dunhill artery forceps 5″ (12.7 cm). It is useful to have a few straight and curved artery forceps of different sizes.
2 Scissors: iris, straight, 4½″; McIndoe's curved 7″ scissors (especially for deeper dissection); 5″ straight, pointed-tip scissors (useful for tissue plane dissection); Metzenbaum straight and curved blunt-tip scissors – of different sizes ('baby' = 4½″ or 6″); Stevens supercut 5⅛″ (13 cm) is an excellent small, flat, curved, pointed-tip pair of scissors.
3 Allis tissue forceps 6″ (15.2 cm).
4 McDonald's dissector (especially useful in carpal tunnel decompression).

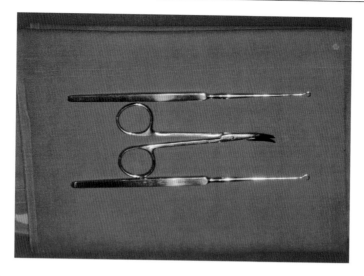

Figure 3.2 Pair of skin hooks and blunt-tip, curved scissors: two important instruments for minor surgery.

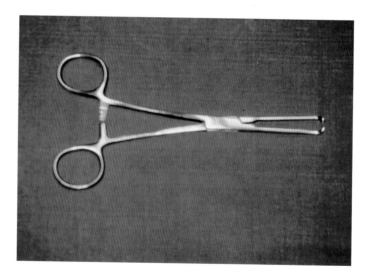

Figure 3.3 Tissue forceps (Allis).

5 Retractors: Kilner, double-ended retractors ('cat's paw retractors')/ small self-retaining retractor.
6 Needle holders: Mayo–Hegar type (6″) or Gillies type are useful additions. The Neivert needle holder (5″) has an ergonomic handle and is good for holding small needles. The Gillies needle holder has no ratchet, and has the scissor incorporated in the instrument.

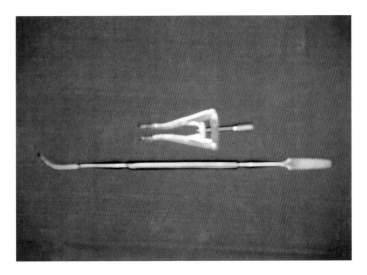

Figure 3.4 Self-retaining retractor (Alm's) and McDonald's dissector.

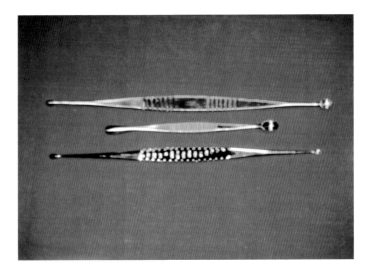

Figure 3.5 Volkmann's double-ended sharp spoon curettes.

7 Curettes: Volkmann double-ended sharp-spoon curette. Usually three (A, B and C) are available. Pre-sterilised disposable ring curettes (e.g. made by Stiefel) are useful.
8 Towel clips (e.g. Backhaus). These are useful if you use surgical drapes for more extensive procedures.
9 Thwaites nail clipper 5⅛″ (13 cm) (Nova Instruments).
10 Nail chisel (Nova Instruments).

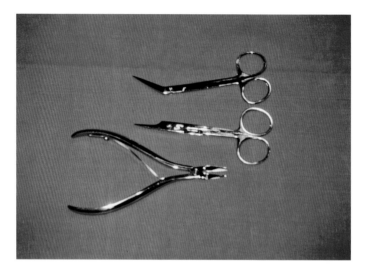

Figure 3.6 Thwaite's nail clipper, straight scissors and Rocket scissors.

Nine and 10 are useful for ingrowing toe-nail (IGTN) surgery, but not essential.

The above list is by no means comprehensive. However, these instruments will easily suffice for the majority of minor surgical procedures. Pre-sterilised, single-use, disposable scalpels and blades, curettes, and punch biopsy instruments are now available at a reasonable price. Further instruments may be required, depending on the type of procedure.

Ingrowing toe-nail

- One scalpel handle, size 3.
- One scalpel blade, size 15.
- One pair of artery forceps, straight 5″ (12.7 cm).
- One pair stitch scissors, sharp/sharp 5″ (12.7 cm), or Thwaites nail clipper (English pattern) 5⅛″ (13 cm) (Nova Instruments), or one Rocket suture scissors (10 cm) (this is a cheaper and excellent alternative to the Thwaites nail clipper).
- One nail chisel (Nova Instruments).
- One Volkmann sharp-spoon curette.
- Wooden applicators with cotton-wool sterile gauze swabs.
- A tourniquet (I use a cut finger of a latex glove, to roll proximally from the tip, which helps to exsanguinate the toe, followed by anchoring with artery forceps). *See* Figure 12.2(a) and (b) on page 196.

Electrocautery

Bleeding and sepsis are the greatest bugbears of surgery. The bleeding encountered during minor surgical procedures can be controlled by pressure, ligation with artery forceps and ligature and electrocautery (from Latin: *cauterium*/Gk: *Kauterion* = to burn with hot iron or caustic substance). Electrocautery is the most useful investment one could make for the provision of minor surgery. It can be used for haemostasis and also for cutting tissues. The great disadvantage is that one cannot control the degree of heat destruction.

The Warecrest C28 cordless cautery is an example of a portable, rechargeable electrocautery, with different types of burners that can be attached to it. Model C28 can use ring cutter, straight cutter, coagulation ball, puncture point and cold point attachments. Their uses are as follows:

- ring and straight cutter: for cutting tissues (e.g. skin tags)
- coagulation ball: for haemostasis of small vessels
- puncture point burner: for releasing subungual haematoma, spider naevi
- cold point burner: ideal for subungual haematoma and spider naevi.

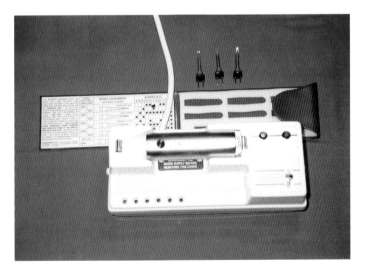

Figure 3.7 C28 with charger and three electrodes.

Cheaper but possibly less durable battery-charged cautery instruments are also available. It is worth looking at instrument catalogues and the Internet before deciding to purchase these.

The hyfrecator

The hyfrecator (e.g. the Birtcher hyfrecator) is more expensive than a C28 but is very useful for extended procedures, such as vasectomies. It has the same function as electrocautery, but one has greater control over the heat generated, compared to the C28 cautery. The hyfrecator can be used for electrofulgaration (Latin: *fulgare* = lightning), electrodessication (Latin: *desiccare* = to dry) and electrocoagulation (Latin: *coagulare* = to curdle).

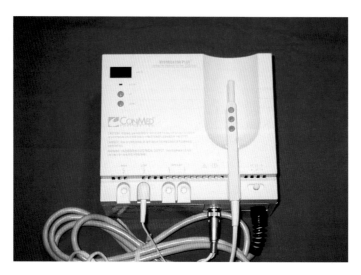

Figure 3.8 Birtcher hyfrecator.

The bipolar mode provides a high-frequency current between the tips of forceps, which provides good coagulation. Its main disadvantage is that it cannot be used for cutting tissues, and the thermal damage caused could be greater, compared to the use of radio waves. Radiosurgical equipment overcomes this, and is more versatile.

Radiosurgical equipment

Radiosurgical instruments work at a much higher frequency than electrosurgical instruments (diathermy), of up to 3.8 MHz. It must be remembered that radiosurgery is not the same as electrosurgery. Unlike the electrode of the hyfrecator, the active electrode in radiosurgery is always 'cold'. Unlike surgical diathermy, the passive plate does not act as an electrode dispersing current, but as a radio antenna, receiving a signal. It need *not* have contact with the patient, and is insulated. When a biterminal radiosurgical instrument is used, the current returns via the patient, and the insulated indifferent or 'ground' plate, which is in reality an *antenna*, helps to focus the radio waves. This allows a greater control of lateral heat. Cell destruction occurs at the tip of the active electrode, due to tissue resistance to the passage of current (known as *impedance*). The active electrode itself does *not* get heated. The effect of the radio wave on the soft tissue produces the surgical result. Different wave forms can be produced by turning a knob, resulting in different surgical effects, including cutting (fully filtered wave form); blend waveform (fully rectified), which cuts and partly coagulates; coag waveform (partially rectified), which only coagulates without cutting; and a FULG or fulguration waveform, which is a spark-gap type and causes superficial tissue destruction with haemostasis. Bipolar coagulation is possible via a suitable cable and insulated forceps.

A useful instrument for primary care is the Ellman DS90 radiosurgery instrument, used by dentists but very useful for minor surgery. This has a power output of 90 watts, which is adequate for use in primary care. The electrodes are autoclavable. Currently a more powerful, 140 watt Ellman Surgitron FFPF is available, with a host of accessories (FFPF is the acronym for fully filtered, fully rectified, partially rectified and fulgaration).

Different types of monopolar electrodes are available, including:

- loop electrodes (round loop, oval loop, diamond loop and triangle loop electrodes of different sizes); used for shave excision, with contouring and planing of lesions

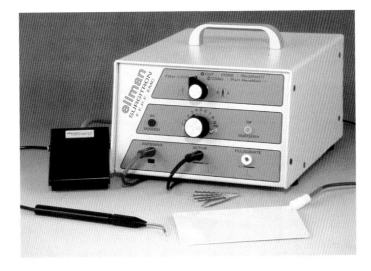

Figure 3.9 The Ellman Surgitron FFPF.

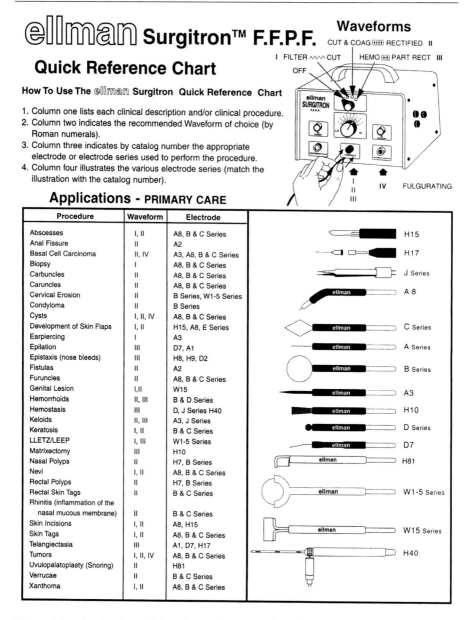

Figure 3.10 Applications of the Ellman Surgitron electrodes in primary care surgery.

- needle electrodes (broad needle, Vari-Tip microdissection needle electrode and fine or regular wire electrodes); broad needle electrodes are used for fulgaration/desiccation or coagulation; the Vari-Tip is composed of adjustable surgical tungsten wire and is used for fine incisions/excisions

- ball electrodes: available in different sizes; used mainly for coagulation, but could also be used for fulgaration/desiccation.

Other special types of electrodes (available for the Ellman Surgitron) include:

- fine, insulated, coated needle electrodes for telangiectasia and epilation (set of three, colour coded)
- matrixectomy electrodes for the destruction of nail matrix, and dealing with nail spicules (set of three).

Special accessories are available for ENT and gynaecological applications.

Radiosurgery is a great advance and is very useful and efficient for many of the primary-care surgical procedures. The types of electrodes, waveform settings and procedures for the Ellman Surgitron are shown in Figure 3.10. The bipolar electrode is an accessory. However, if coagulation of a small artery is needed, the artery could be grasped with a mosquitoe forceps, and coagulation effected by touching the handle of the forceps with the monopolar electrode. The terms monopolar and bipolar are conventionally used to denote the number of active electrodes contacting the tissues. Thus, a coagulating forceps with the two tips touching the tissue is a bipolar forceps. Monoterminal and biterminal denote the method of delivery of the current. An example of monoterminal delivery is the hyfrecator, when it is used without the indifferent electrode. In radiosurgery equipment, fulguration is effected by monoterminal means, since the antenna plate is unnecessary for electrofulgaration/desiccation. Cutting, cutting/coagulation and coagulation are biterminal procedures.

Contraindications for radiosurgery

PATIENT
- It is best to avoid patients with cardiac pacemakers for operations in a primary-care setting, where an anaesthetist is not available. These patients are best operated on in hospital settings.
- Gaseous bowel distension, in a highly constipated patient. This could be dangerous especially if you are working on lesions around the perineum. There is a potential for explosion since bowel gases are highly flammable.
- Avoid using alcohol for skin cleansing. If you do, ensure that the surface is wiped dry, preferably after using a saline or Savlon® swab.

SURGEON
If you have unsteady hands! Radiosurgery requires fine, steady movements of the fingers and wrists. This can be helped by steadying the wrist

and distal forearm on the patient, near the area of surgery. As in micro-vascular surgery, it is advisable not to have any stimulants, such as alcohol, for at least 12–24 hours before operating. Alcohol is known to induce tremors in most individuals!

If you are purchasing and using this equipment, it is strongly advised that you familiarise yourself with the theory of radiosurgery, and practise with the instrument, ideally under supervision. It is important to learn the technique of handling the different electrodes and the power settings in your operating room environment, as environmental temperature, ventila-tion, and the presence of other radio waves (e.g. having music on while operating) have an effect on the efficacy of the instrument, which could be optimised using the power settings. The after-care of the reusable elec-trode is important. Although the electrodes can be steam sterilised, chemical sterilisation is known to be less damaging to the insulating rubber. Strict adherence to the manufacturer's guidelines for electrosurgical safety, given in their 'safety and warnings' sheet, is very important. It is important to practise, using the various electrodes, on a fresh, moist piece of steak. The radiosurgical method of incisions and excisions are a contrast to scalpel incisions, which need pressure. The technique in radiosurgery requires a mastery of gentle, non-pressure movements, an artistry that needs practice.

It is important to remember that the lateral heat produced is directly proportional to the size (S) of the electrode (the finer the electrode, the lesser the lateral heat), the wave (W) form (minimal in cutting, and maximal in fulgaration), intensity (I) of current (controlled by the power setting) and time (T) of contact with the tissue. It is inversely proportional to the frequency of the current (3.8 MHz in the Ellman Surgitron) and impedance (Imp) of the tissue.

$$\text{Lateral heat} = \frac{S \times W \times I \times T}{F \times \text{Imp}}$$

In addition to the seven standard electrodes that come with the equip-ment, three useful accessories from the primary-care perspective are:

1   The bipolar forceps, which enables more precise haemostasis.
2   Insulated matrix electrodes set (three electrodes: a 2 mm, 4 mm and a nail-spicule electrode).
3   Insulated sclerotherapy needle set. (Needle gauge: 0.004, white insu-lation; 0.007, violet insulation; and 0.009, orange insulation. All three needles have a 1/16 shaft. A 3/32 shaft needle set has a differ-ent colour code.) These needles have other uses, such as epilation. The manufacturers include excellent instructions on use and care with each set.

Cryo-equipment

Commonly used cryogens are:

- Liquid nitrogen – via a cotton-wool swab applicator, cryospray or cryoprobe. Boils at –196°C (Cry-AC®, Cryo-tec® or CryoPro®). The static holding time depends on the size of the equipment. A 350 ml volume has a holding time of about 12 hours; and a 500 ml volume has a holding time of about 24 hours.
- Dimethyl-ether and propane aerosol (Histofreezer). Useful for thin, benign lesions; reaches a temperature of about –57°C. If used on warts, you need to pare down the wart before application of the cryogen. It has a long shelf-life and is relatively cheaper.

The following are not commonly used in primary care:

- Nitrous oxide as a cryoprobe.
- Carbon dioxide snow.

Liquid nitrogen must be stored in special flasks called Storage Dewars which vary in capacity and storage times.

Sterilisers

It is only when they go wrong that machines remind you how powerful they are.

Clive James

Sterilisation is the destruction of all living organisms. *Disinfection* is the *reduction* of a population of pathogenic micro-organisms without achieving sterility. Not all bacterial spores are destroyed.

There are five methods of sterilising or disinfecting instruments in general practice.

1 Antiseptic solutions.
2 Boiling. Bacterial spores and some viruses are resistant. Used when access to superior sterilisation is not available (in rural areas of developing countries).
3 Hot-air ovens (hardly used in primary care). They are cheaper than autoclaves, but take longer to sterilise. The Medi-Clave Hot Air Steriliser and Memmert Hot Air Steriliser are examples.

4   Non-vacuum and vacuum autoclaves (saturated steam under pressure).
5   Use of CSSD facilities.

One of the most serious infections is hepatitis B or serum hepatitis, which may be transmitted from patient to patient by as little as 0.0001 ml of infected blood. The virus remains active for up to 6 months in dried blood; consequently instruments that have been poorly cleaned or disinfected may be responsible for infecting other patients, while poor surgical technique may result in the doctor becoming infected from the patient.

Sterilisation and not disinfection should be the aim of every surgery. In practice this means autoclaving or using dry-heat ovens for the majority of items.

Autoclaves

Autoclaving achieves sterilisation by using *saturated steam*. It is the most efficient way of sterilising instruments, packs and dressings. An autoclave is basically a pressure cooker. A domestic pressure cooker could also be used to sterilise instruments.

Two types of bench-top steam autoclaves are used in primary care:

* conventional non-vacuum autoclaves
* vacuum autoclaves.

The conventional autoclaves depend on the passive displacement of air from the chamber as the steam pressure increases prior to the sterilisation cycle. They can only be used for sterilising unwrapped instruments. They are not efficient for sterilising complex instruments with cavities or internal lumina, as there is a theoretical danger of pockets of contaminated air becoming trapped therein, reducing the efficacy of steam penetration. Non-vacuum autoclaves can be used for sterilising solid instruments for immediate use. The instruments must be heat sensitive.

Vacuum autoclaves have the advantage of being useful for the sterilisation of instruments in paper pouches, textile products, wrapped cassettes or instruments that have a lumen. Solid instruments can be sterilised for aseptic storage with a view to usage at a later time. The sterilisation cycle is preceded by a phase when a vacuum pump extracts the air contained within both the chamber and the instrument load. An equalisation phase at the end of the sterilisation phase results in the chamber pressure normalising, allowing the door to be opened.

Most autoclaves are provided with a printer/recorder, allowing a permanent record of every cycle. The *'CE' mark*, indicating compliance with the Medical Devices Directive 93/42/EEC, became mandatory in the

United Kingdom in June 1998. Purchase only autoclaves that have a 'CE' mark. Efficient sterilisation involves:

- frequent performance checks
- regular inspections
- maintenance.

The Medical Devices Agency, which is an executive agency of the Department of Health in the UK, has published two Device Bulletins giving information about bench-top sterilisers. They are: *The Purchase, Operation and Maintenance of Bench-top Sterilisers* (DB9605) and *The Validation and Periodic Testing of Bench-top Vacuum Steam Sterilisers* (DB9804). These documents provide useful information for those contemplating the purchase of steam sterilisers.

Temperature, pressure and sterilising time:

- 'quick' cycle, 134°C (273°F) for 3.5 min under a pressure of 30 lbf/in^2 (207 kPa).

The main disadvantage of the smaller non-vacuum autoclave is that instrument packs cannot be sterilised as there is not a vacuum cycle to extract air and dry the packs.

Whichever steriliser is chosen, it is important that it is regularly *checked* and *serviced*. It would be wise to ask for a demonstration before purchasing. It is important to organise a maintenance contract at the time of purchase.

Distilled water should be used in the autoclave to reduce the deposition of chalk and solids within the sterilising chamber and on the heating element.

As mentioned earlier, a steriliser is not an instrument washer: *it is essential that all instruments are scrubbed clean in warm, soapy water and rinsed before being sterilised.* Particles of dirt or secretions or blood may be baked on the surface of the instrument, especially the crevices as in box joints and in serrations. Then sterility may not be guaranteed. Special brush sets (each brush has more bristles per square inch) are available to clean them manually, reducing the possibility of damaging the instruments and leading to corrosion.

Ultrasonic cleansing equipment is also available. This will save time for the practice nurse, is useful for hollow instruments, and will be cost-effective if many procedures are done in a session or a whole day. Ultrasonic cleansing equipment comes in small, medium and large sizes. Ultrasonic cleaning agents or multi-enzymatic cleaning solutions are used, and the temperature and duration can be regulated in the equipment that comes with heaters. However, one needs to be aware of the purchasing and maintenance costs for this equipment. For the average practice doing a few procedures a day, or doing mainly cutaneous and subcutaneous surgery, the chance of being left with very dirty instruments with blood and fat is very unlikely.

Under normal circumstances decontamination procedures may be defined in terms of temperature and time, and may be summarised as follows:[1]

- saturated steam (e.g. autoclaving)
     2.2 bar (0.22 mPa) pressure at 121°C for 15 min or 134°C for 3 min
- dry heat (e.g. hot-air ovens; equipment utilising dry heat is hardly used nowadays in the UK)
     160°C for 60 min holding time or 180°C for 30 min
- boiling water (hot water disinfects)
     98–100°C for a minimum of 5 min. For decontamination of equipment, linen or other surfaces contaminated with hepatitis B or HIV.

Hot-water disinfection or other boiling methods are *not* preferred techniques, as in practice it is difficult to monitor the decontamination temperature and time cycle. Boiling water will not kill bacterial spores. It cannot be used for decontaminating items that are required to have been sterilised (i.e. those instruments that go into sterile body areas) such as surgical scissors, forceps, stitch cutters and uterine sounds. However, this method is still used in some rural areas of developing countries, when there is no access to sterilisers. There is no reason why at least a pressure cooker cannot be used under these circumstances.

General practitioners who contemplate the installation of a portable steam steriliser will need to consider carefully the use to which they will put the equipment.

Use of CSSD

If you have access to the local hospital CSSD, it may be cost-effective to acquire sterilised instruments and towels, or minor surgery sets personalised to your instructions for your minor surgery sessions. It is worth negotiating the costs with the CSSD and working out details of transport of sets to and from the practice.

Pre-packed disposable sterile instruments

Increasing numbers of disposable sterile instruments are available in the catalogues. These are very helpful for use in high-risk patients (hepatitis B positive or HIV positive). They are also very effective in preventing cross-infection. They are convenient, in obviating the need for sterilisation by the nurse, saving time. Examples of useful disposable instruments are the *ring curettes* and *biopsy punch* instruments available from Stiefel. The Stiefel ring curettes come in two ring sizes (4 mm or 7 mm). They are sold in boxes of ten. The biopsy punches have a punch size of 2 mm, 3 mm, 4 mm, 5 mm, 6 mm and 8 mm. Bearing in mind that the majority of cutaneous lesions excised by general practitioners are less than 10 mm diameter, these instruments are convenient to use in primary care. The disposable biopsy punch also comes in boxes of ten.

Antiseptic solutions

Traditionally 70% alcohol was the most widely used antiseptic solution, subsequently with the addition of 0.5% chlorhexidine. This is widely used for emergency disinfection of surgical instruments, requiring only 2 minutes' immersion. Where instruments are left for longer periods or stored continuously, the addition of one tablet of sodium nitrite BPC 1 gram will prevent rusting. As the tablet dissolves over several days, another is added. It is recommended that all instruments used in minor surgery are sterilised using autoclaves.

Indeed, above all else, a wound must be made clean.
Theodoric (1205–1296)

Resuscitation equipment

The majority of minor operations will be done under local anaesthetic, which is mostly safe. Problems may arise from inappropriate choice of patients, e.g. operating on patients with associated illnesses such as cardiac dysrhythmias.

However, it is useful to have resuscitation facilities and to be familiar with their use and to update and check them regularly. The following items should be included where possible:

1 airway support and ventilation devices (minimum requirement); selection of plastic airways (Guedel airways) or Brook airway/Laerdal pocket mask and valve (essential or minimum requirement)
2 drugs such as adrenaline, hydrocortisone, atropine and chlorpheniramine (essential or minimum requirement)
3 large selection of syringes and needles (essential)

  4 positive-pressure inflator (Ambu) (desirable)
  5 endotracheal tubes (desirable)
  6 laryngoscope (desirable – check batteries periodically!)
  7 suction apparatus (desirable – hand operated, e.g. Vitalograph or electrical)
  8 intravenous cannulae
  9 giving sets for intravenous fluids
10 oxygen cylinders and giving sets
11 Entonox®
12 ECG machine
13 cardiac defibrillator.

Items 1, 2 and 3 must be available and are *essential* items in any surgery; 4–7 are *desirable*, especially if procedures such as sclerotherapy and intravenous anaesthesia are used; 8–13 are *ideal*. One has to weigh the extremely low risk of major anaphylaxis against the cost of acquiring and maintaining equipment like a defibrillator. However, in large rural practices it would be useful equipment to have – for resuscitation of patients, arresting after an infarct – where transfer to a hospital would take time.

    All doctors, nurses and practice staff should be proficient in basic life support skills. Skills in advanced life support are useful for all doctors who work in rural settings, where very quick access to an ambulance crew or BASICS team is not available.

Entonox®

Entonox® (50% nitrous oxide, 50% oxygen) with mask and giving set is a most useful item in any treatment room. It is very useful for children, and is an excellent pain reliever. Recovery is almost immediate on stopping, without hangover. Being an anaesthetic, Entonox® may be included for reimbursement under paragraph 44 of the *Red Book*.

Magnifiers

Magnification has two main uses. They are useful for diagnosis, and for operation on small lesions and tissue. It is extremely useful to have magnifiers available for the assessment of cutaneous lesions. If used regularly, they could enhance the diagnostic accuracy of the user. Illuminated magnifiers are available commercially. Magnifications of ×2, ×3, ×10 or ×30 are used. The *Dermatoscope* is an instrument that is used increasingly by doctors dealing with pigmented cutaneous lesions, for

enhancing diagnostic skills. It is useful for the early diagnosis of pigmented skin lesions such as malignant melanoma. It utilises 2.5 V halogen
illumination and magnifies the lesion which has been moistened with
olive or paraffin oil to ×10, and allows the user to measure the size of
the lesion in millimetres, since the contact glass is marked with a scale. It
can be used for skin surface microscopy of a lesion. The Dermatoscope
costs around £300. This standard magnification and illumination has
enabled doctors to do research into its diagnostic usefulness, and compare results internationally. Experience in this science of *epiluminescence
microscopy* (ELM) has enabled practitioners to enhance their clinical
diagnostic accuracy.[2] Its main use lies in the diagnosis of melanocytic
and non-melanocytic lesions, and then proceeding to distinguish between
benign and malignant melanocytic lesions, using the ABCD rule of dermatoscopy[3] derived from the original ABCD rule described by Friedman for
the early clinical detection of malignant melanoma. Included in the Heine
Dermatoscope kit is a useful compendium for differential diagnosis of
pigmented lesions.

Magnification loupes

Magnification loupes are available which can be worn with spectacles,
and provide sufficient magnification to work comfortably; some also
have illumination. Usually ×2.5 magnification allows the surgeon to
operate on very small lesions or very fine blood vessels, and to use very
fine sutures. For example, loupe magnification will be useful for treating
telangiectases with radiosurgery fine electrodes.

Ultraviolet (Wood's light)

Various instruments producing fluorescent ultraviolet A light are used
to assess skin lesions. They are especially useful for clinical diagnosis of
fungal skin infections.

Other equipment and materials

Cotton wool on 'orange sticks', spirit swabs, dental pledgets (for sclerotherapy of varicose veins), various types and sizes of plasters, contact
wound dressings, skin markers, adhesive tapes and conforming bandages
are other items that should be available in a treatment room. The practice

nurse is the appropriate person for taking stock and ensuring that they are available.

Digital photography

Excellent digital cameras are currently available. High-resolution digital images are very useful for the remote sharing of clinical signs with colleagues or specialists, especially to get a second opinion from any part of the world. Digital images are also useful for keeping graphic records of pre-treatment and post-treatment appearances. They are an excellent teaching and learning tool. For example, it is possible to store the image of a cutaneous lesion in a computer as a file and send it by electronic mail to a specialist for a second opinion; or to store it in the patient's record. The prices of digital cameras are decreasing and soon they will be an affordable purchase. They can also provide useful evidence when medico-legal problems arise post-operatively.

Waste disposal

- Sharps disposal – approved container, incinerated.
- Clinical waste disposal – yellow bag, incinerated.
- General waste disposal – black plastic bag, sent to landfill sites for burial.

Adequate arrangements are required for the disposal of 'sharps' and clinical waste such as dressings. Each health authority has procedures for dealing with contaminated 'sharps' and most general practitioners now have 'bins' for storing needles, blades and other sharp objects, which are destroyed by incineration when three-quarters full. In the United Kingdom, the Family Health Services Authority offers a waste-disposal service. **Gloves must be worn by all staff handling sharps and swabs with body fluids (blood, exudates).**

Beware!

During preparation, operation and post-operative disposal of materials:

EVERY PATIENT IS POTENTIALLY INFECTED!
PROTECT YOURSELF!

Clinical waste disposal (human tissue, body fluids, drugs, swabs) must be in a *yellow* plastic bag, sealed, source identified and incinerated. The Health and Safety Act of 1974 states that it is the responsibility of the employer to ensure the safe disposal of waste, and that all staff are aware of waste management.

General waste disposal will be in *black* plastic bags. These are very often removed by the cleaners.

Some useful Internet resources

It is worth searching the web for the product you wish to purchase. This can be done through any search engine. The following are useful search engines:

Altavista	*www.altavista.digital.com*
Yahoo	*www.yahoo.com*
Infoseek	*www.infoseek.com*
Excite	*www.excite.com*
Lycos	*www.lycos.com*

Personally, I prefer altavista, as it seems to be faster. I would recommend that you try all initially. The following are the web sites for the Ellman Surgitron and Histofreezer:

* *www.ellman.com*
* *www.histofreezer.com*

References

1   DHSS. *AIDS: Guidance for Surgeons, Anaesthetists, Dentists and their Teams Dealing with Patients Infected with HIV.* Booklet 3. London, DHSS; 1986.

2   Steiner A, Pehamberger H and Wolff K. *In vivo* epiluminescence microscopy of pigmented lesions. II Diagnosis of small pigmented lesions and early detection of malignant melanoma. *J Am Acad Dermatol.* 1987; **17**: 584–91.

3   Nachbar F, Stolz W, Merkle T *et al.* The ABCD rule of dermatoscopy. *J Am Acad Dermatol.* 1994; **30**(4): 551–9.

Further reading

British Medical Association. *A Code of Practice for Sterilisation of Instruments and Control of Cross Infection*. London, BMA; 1989.

British Medical Association. *A Code of Practice for the Safe Use and Disposal of Sharps*. London, BMA; 1990.

Brown JS. *Minor Surgery. A Text and Atlas* (3e). London, Chapman & Hall; 1997.

Pollack VS. *Electrosurgery of the Skin*. New York, Churchill Livingstone; 1991.

4

The role of the practice nurse in minor surgery

The trained nurse has become one of the greatest blessings of humanity, taking a place beside the surgeon and the patient, and not inferior to either in her mission.

Sir William Osler (1849–1919)

Overview

- Role of practice nurse in minor surgery:
  - equipment and instrument maintenance
  - drug stock-keeping
  - organisational
  - surgical
  - extended role of practice nurse
- Infection control:
  - staff protection
  - patient protection
- Administration
- Guidelines for good practice in minor surgery.

Role of the practice nurse

The help of a nurse for minor surgery, especially for excision of lesions and sclerotherapy, is invaluable. Being a very useful member of the clinical team, it is important to liaise with the practice nurse who will assist you in your procedures. It is useful to discuss your needs for the various procedures, and it is important for the nurse to be aware of your requirements. The well-organised surgical team will be effective and efficient.

The nurse's duties will include the following.

- Liaison with administrative staff – regarding date, time, details of patients and procedures.
- Ensuring that all equipment required for the operations is available, including sterilisation of instruments.
- Checking whether written consent is required and has been taken prior to the operation.
- Preparation of the trolley with instruments.
- Counselling the patient.
- Liaison with the surgeon, pre-operatively, especially on the day of the minor surgery list. The nurse may need to clarify whether any special instruments need to be sterilised, or equipment set up. Having a written list of instruments required by the surgeon for specific procedures is useful, especially if more than one partner is doing minor surgery. Assisting at operation if needed. Checking the local anaesthetic *with the surgeon*, especially to confirm whether it is the correct drug and the date of expiry, is a very important function of the nurse. This double checking prevents the possibility of using the wrong drug or an outdated drug, an area for litigation which is not uncommon.
- Post-operatively, ensuring that sharps have been disposed appropriately by the surgeon, and cleaning and sterilising the instruments. It is good practice for the surgeon to dispose of all sharps, including blades and needles, which is his responsibility. This prevents needle-stick injuries to the nurse.
- Applying dressings post-operatively, advice, and giving any post-operative written instructions.
- Paperwork:
  - checking whether the surgeon has written the operative notes;
  - checking whether the pathology specimen bottle has been adequately labelled and the histopathology form filled;
  - logging procedure in the minor ops book/computer;
  - giving patient a follow-up appointment to see a nurse/doctor;
  - write FP10 for PPA, and get surgeon to sign.

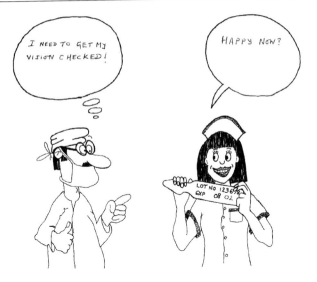

Figure 4.1 Doctor and nurse with ampoule.

- The nurse should liaise with the surgeon if any post-operative wound complications occur. Complications need to be documented for audit purposes.
- Removing sutures at appropriate time. Liase with the surgeon if needed. It is important to ensure that the nurse is competent in the science and art of removing sutures.
- Maintaining audit data.
- Checking every month whether the histology reports have arrived, and have been checked by the surgeon. If not, check with hospital.

More important than the technical artistry of the surgeon is the tender loving care with professionalism provided by the nurse. He/she nurtures the patient into a person. It is therefore the surgeon's responsibility to train nurses adequately.

Reflections

- Have you observed your nurse removing sutures after surgical procedures?
- Is he/she familiar with different types of suture materials, methods of suturing, knots and healing times in different anatomical areas of the body?

Potential extended role for the practice nurse

In some settings, a further extended role for the nurse has been identified. Nurses with appropriate knowledge and experience can be trained in specific procedures, which they can undertake with or without supervision. Some examples of extended roles are:

- suturing of lacerations
- cryotherapy for warts.

There are two important issues to consider:

Medico-legal issues

The crucial skill is the clinical assessment and diagnosis of wounds and lesions. Clear guidelines will be available from the nursing organisations on this.

Diagnostic and technical skills

The nurse who undertakes the role of making an initial assessment and management of the patient, without any medical practitioner involvement, should not only have the confidence, but also the competence and ability to deal with unexpected outcomes during the procedure. In some settings, the nurse makes an initial assessment of a patient following an injury, considers it a 'minor injury' and manages the patient. It must be remembered that no injury is 'minor' to the patient. Though the apparent force or mechanism that caused the injury may be 'minor', we can classify it as 'minor' only after a clinical examination and diagnosis. From the doctor's perspective it may be considered 'minor' when the condition is self-limiting, hardly leads to complications and can be managed with simple analgesics and self-care.

The level of involvement and the degree of responsibility will depend on the medico-legal issues and the nurse's employing practitioner. A nurse who has had training in suturing technique and giving local anaesthetic could undertake the suturing of superficial wounds *after* the assessment and diagnosis by the doctor. In this situation, the ultimate responsibility lies with the doctor, and the trained nurse with the appropriate technical skill undertakes the suturing and care of the wound. This is not uncommon in rural settings, where a nearby casualty or emergency unit is not available.

If the nurse acts as an autonomous practitioner, making the diagnosis, assessment and proceeding to manage, it is very important to ensure that such a person has been adequately trained, and officially accredited to do so. The training obviously is more extensive – including a curriculum which incorporates anatomy, physiology, pathology, pharmacology and technical training in models, animal tissues and supervised suturing, with awareness of all potential pitfalls, their prevention and management, prior to accreditation. The same applies for treating warts. In many wart clinics run in secondary-care settings, a dermatologist makes the clinical diagnosis and assessment, followed by the nurse/nurse practitioner treating by cryotherapy. This requires only the technical skill of using cryotherapy, and the training required is less intensive, and cost-effective.

Infection control

When I look upon the past, I can only dispel the sadness which falls upon me by gazing into that happy future when the infection will be banished … The conviction that such a time must inevitably sooner or later arrive will cheer my dying hour.

Ignaz Semmelweis (1818–1865)

Staff protection

Doctors and nurses undertaking minor surgery should be actively immunised against hepatitis B. Active immunisation involves *three doses* of hepatitis B vaccine (e.g. Engerix B® or H-B-Vax®). The dosage for adults is 20 µg (1.0 ml). The second dose is given after 4 weeks, and the third 6 months after the first dose. An antibody level of 100 miu/ml is considered to be protective. Antibody titres should be checked 2–4 months after completion of immunisation. This confers an immunity for at least 3–5 years. Healthcare staff should receive **boosters every 3–5 years** after the primary course. The policies followed by staff for the prevention of hepatitis B will be effective in preventing HIV infection. Currently, immunisation against hepatitis A and B viruses (HAV, HBV) are available as combined vaccines. The Department of Health guidelines define *exposure-prone procedure* (EPP) as one in which there is a risk of injury to the healthcare worker from exposure to the patient's open tissues. These include those procedures where the gloved hand or finger tips of the healthcare worker are not completely visible at *all times*, by virtue of it being in a patient's body cavity or deep wound, or confined anatomical space. A healthcare worker who is either HIV or hepatitis B-antigen positive must *not* perform such procedures. Internal examinations or procedures that do not require the use of sharp instruments are not considered to be EPP.

It is useful to highlight, by documenting in the summary sheet of patient notes, if the individual is hepatitis B virus (HBV), hepatitis C virus (HCV) or human immune deficiency virus (HIV) positive. This will warn the clinical staff towards being more cautious. If clinical records are held electronically, ensure that the information is available in the morbidity summary page.

Protection during procedures can be achieved by the wearing of gloves (and double gloves for high-risk procedures) and correct handling of sharps – especially needles and scalpels.

Remember

EVERY PATIENT IS POTENTIALLY INFECTED!
PROTECT YOURSELF!

Protection of the patient

The *ten commandments* of patient protection from any infection are:

1 adequate skin preparation
2 aseptic and antiseptic technique (sterile gloves)
3 use of prophylactic antibiotics when needed
4 gentle handling of tissues
5 adequate haemostasis
6 avoiding tension when closing incisions
7 avoiding dead space when closing incisions
8 appropriate apposition of wound edges
9 surgeon should avoid operating if he has a 'cold', septic lesion or open wound in the hand
10 use of sterile dressings.

Administration

*We trained very hard, but it seemed that every time we were begin-
ning to form up into teams, we would be reorganised. I was to learn
later in life that we tend to meet any new situation by reorganising,
and a wonderful method it can be for creating the illusion of progress!*
Caius Petronius (AD 66)

The practice team must be fully aware of the procedures and protocol for
minor surgery in their own practice.

At consultation

A decision is made with the patient regarding the time, date and place of
surgery, depending on the nature of the problem. Injections are usually
carried out during consultations or at another 'double appointment'
booked at a more convenient date. Excision of lesions is usually done on
a separate date, in the treatment room – as a planned procedure, with the
assistance of the nurse.

Pre-operative assessment

This includes a clinical diagnosis of the *site* and *nature* of the lesion,
explanation to the patient about the treatment options and a shared plan
of management. A useful checklist includes the following.

- What is the *site* and *nature* (anatomical and histological diagnosis) of
  the lesion?
- Is the patient '*fit*' for the procedure to be carried out in primary care?
  (Have you considered the patient's anxieties, allergies and associated
  illnesses?)
- Have you *explained* the *procedure* and possible *outcomes*?
- Have you obtained written *consent* for surgery? (Your procedure may
  be to get the written consent on the day of the surgery.)
- Is the *nurse* aware of the date, time and nature of the procedure? (Best
  documented in the nurse's book.) The receptionist/admin staff need to
  document the date/time and patient particulars in the appointment

register or separate minor op book – depending on the practice. It is useful to give the patient a written card documenting the date and time for minor surgery. The card will be useful to document follow-up dates to see the nurse and doctor. Some patients tend to forget!

- Any *instructions* to the patient regarding preparation for surgery (e.g. shower before coming to the surgery/prophylactic antibiotics if indicated)?

Operation day

- Are the necessary instruments and agents required for the procedure sterilised and laid out? (Usually the nurse's responsibility, although the surgeon needs to double check.)
- Are the specimen bottles and histology forms available and labelled?
- Have you obtained consent?
- Have you *counselled* the patient on what you are going to do?

Post-operative administration

- Have the histology forms and specimen bottles been appropriately completed and labelled?
- Have you given appropriate post-operative instructions to the patient? (Verbal or written, such as analgesia and what to look for.)
- Does the patient need a prescription for any analgesics or other medications?
- Has a follow-up appointment to see the nurse and the doctor been given to the patient – written on the card? Usually the patient sees the nurse for removal of sutures. The doctor usually sees at 4 weeks, when the histology report will be available and a post-operative scar check can be done.
- Are all the details of the procedure documented in the *operations register*/separate A5 minor op card or computer database? Coding for the procedures is useful for audit (*see* Appendices A and B).
- Has the nurse ensured that the doctor has signed the FP10 for the materials used, which needs to be sent to the PPA?
- Does the nurse or administrative staff check the operations book at least *monthly*, to ensure that the histology results have arrived. If they have not arrived, who will do the 'chasing up' with the hospital?

Summary of administration

Ensure that an appointment system, consent form (especially for removal of lesions), operations register and a follow-up system are in operation. If you do not have the above systems in operation, it is worth organising them for the future as they are a reflection of the quality of management.

Reflections

- Is it mandatory to get *written* consent from the patient?

- What is your practice policy?

- When will you deviate from it?

Management of specimens

Most of the administrative work and management of specimens could be delegated to the practice nurse.

All specimens must be sent for histology, to confirm the pre-operative clinical and histological diagnosis. It must be remembered that the final diagnosis of any lesion is histological. Specimens are usually sent in 10% formol-saline, with the specimen bottle labelled to identify the patient. The appropriate forms should be filled, giving all the requested information that is necessary for the pathologist reporting on the specimen.

Reflections

- Will you send an obvious skin tag (benign fibroepithelioma) for histology?

  By obvious I mean the filiform small skin tags. Sessile lesions may turn out to be an intradermal naevus.

  (I explain to the patient – and let the patient decide! I also offer the specimen in formaline for the patient to keep if he/she wishes!)

  Whatever the choice of the patient, document it in the notes.

Guidelines for good practice in minor surgery

Guidelines are not goal lines!

Responsibility: surgeon= S; nurse= N; cleaners= C.

- Ensure that all staff are fully aware about the control of infection against HBV, and ideally immune to HBV infection. It is good policy to have a record of their immunisation status. (S,N)
- Ensure that all staff handling body fluids or blood are fully aware of the potential risk of infection and take adequate barrier precautions, such as wearing gloves. (S,N)
- Sterile gloves should be worn by the surgeon and assistant, when removing lesions. (S,N)
- Alternatives to latex should be used by staff allergic to latex. Biogel® and Allegard® are two examples of alternative surgical gloves. (S,N)
- The surgeon and assistant should wear plastic aprons when removing deep lesions where there is a likelihood of blood spillage. (S,N)
- Mask and eye protection may be required if there is a risk of spray from body fluids. Goggles should be readily available if there is a high likelihood of spray or plumes from electrocautery. (S,N)
- Work surfaces should be cleaned before and after minor surgery. 1 : 1000 parts household bleach or alcohol wipes should be used. (N)
- If blood spillage has occurred, clean using neat household bleach or hot water and detergent, then rinse with disposable wipes. Thick rubber gloves should be worn. (N)
- Instruments need to be sterilised by autoclaving or dry heat immediately prior to use, unless sterilised in pouches by vacuum autoclaves. (N)
- Leave instruments in autoclave/steriliser until just before use. (N)
- Cover instruments before use with sterile towel (use it within 3 hours). (N)
- After use, clean instruments with hot water and detergent while wearing gloves, then sterilise. Ultrasound cleansing equipment is useful if many procedures are done in one session and hollow tubular instruments are used. (N)
- Specimens for histopathology should be placed directly into the appropriate sample container. (S,N)
- After covering with formaldehyde, they should be sealed and labelled. (N)
- Syringe needles, anaesthetic needles and blades should be put in a sharps container after use, to reduce the risk of a sharps injury when clearing away. (S,N)

- Clinical waste must be put into pedal bins, lined with a yellow bag, in each consulting room. (N)
- These bins should be emptied after each surgery. (N)
- Yellow bags have 'For Incineration' marked clearly on the outside. (N)
- General waste is disposed of in black bags. (N)
- Waste awaiting collection should be stored in a well-drained, hard standing area, which can be washed down. (N,C)
- This storage area should not be accessible to unauthorised persons. It should be safe from animals, vermin and insects. (C)
- Aerosols, glass and batteries should be put into cardboard boxes and sealed. (N)
- Sharps containers should be locked and sealed when three-quarters full. Do NOT store inside any bag. Store separately from other clinical waste. (N)
- Clinical waste should show the surgery identification before leaving the practice. (N)

Guidelines are guidelines and not protocols.

From the perspective of health and safety of the staff, it is important to have a protocol in every practice to deal with sharps injuries and contamination of skin and/or mucous membranes from infected or potentially infected blood or body fluids. This is an important area of risk management in primary care. Previous surveys[1,2] have shown that about half the doctors in general practices surveyed did not know or were unsure about the risk from needlestick injuries, and over half did not have a practice policy for controlling infection. Local guidance or guidelines may exist. It is useful to contact the local Public Health Unit or Consultant for Communicable Disease Control in your area. Based on these communications you may wish to write up your practice protocol for dealing with sharps injuries and potential risk exposures by staff. The practice manager could implement this. The protocol should include immediate notification to a responsible person, first aid actions, documentation of details of the incident on the exposed person's file or a separate register (immune status of exposed person, when, where and how of exposure, what material and details of source of exposure). A documented management plan must be operational in your practice. Do you have an 'incident book' in the practice?

An excellent booklet published by the Department of Health (DoH), called *Guidance for Clinical Health Care Workers: Protection from Infection with Blood-borne Viruses*, is now available. The contents are taken from the recommendations of the Expert Advisory Group on AIDS and the Advisory Group on Hepatitis. It is also available on the DoH's website at *http://www.open.gov.uk/doh/chcguid1.htm*

Reflections

- Do you have a practice protocol for infection control, including staff protection?

- What actions are implemented if a practice nurse sustains a needlestick injury?

- Who is responsible for the monitoring, maintenance and stock-taking of equipment and instruments?

- What is an exposure-prone procedure?

References

1   Foy C, Gallagher M, Rhodes T *et al*. HIV and measures to control infection in general practice. *BMJ*. 1990; **300**(6731): 1048–9.

2   White RR and Smith JM. Infection control in general practice: results of a questionnaire survey. *J Pub Hlth Med*. 1995; **17**(2): 146–9.

Further reading

British Medical Association. *A Code of Practice for Sterilisation of Instruments and Control of Cross Infection*. London, BMA; 1989.

British Medical Association. *A Code of Practice for the Safe Use and Disposal of Sharps*. London, BMA; 1990.

Davis PA, Corless DJ and Wastell C. Hazards from surgical gloves. (Letter) *Ann RCS England*. 1997; **79**(6): 467–8.

Department of Health. *Guidance for Clinical Health Care Workers: Protection from Infection with Blood-borne Viruses*. London, HMSO; 1998.

This booklet gives excellent guidance on the prevention and management of BBV infections for HCWs, and covers all the clinical and legal issues (website address: www.open.gov.uk/doh/chcguid1.htm)

Ellis H. Hazards from surgical gloves. (Review) *Ann RCS England.* 1997; **79**(3): 161–3.

Evans TR (ed.) *ABC of Resuscitation* (3e). London, British Medical Association; 1995.

Hoffman P *et al.* Control of infection in general practice: a survey and recommendations. *BMJ.* 1988; **297**: 34–6.

Joint Working Party. Risks to surgeons and patients from HIV and hepatitis: guidelines on precaution and management of exposure to blood or body fluids. *BMJ.* 1992; **305**: 1337–43.

Kiernan M. Minor surgery in general practice: avoiding the pitfalls. *Community Nurse.* 1997; **3**(10): 50–1.

Pollack VS. *Electrosurgery of the Skin.* New York, Churchill Livingstone; 1991.

Appendix A Manual record of minor surgery with recommended procedure codes

1 NAME AND NHS NO.	2 ADDRESS/ TEL	3 DATE OF BIRTH	4 DATE OF OPERATION	5 PROCEDURE CODE*	6 INDICATION	7 HISTO SPECIMEN	8 RESULTS	9 F/U AND COMMENTS	10 SURGEON

* I = INJ
A = ASP
N = INCISION
E = EXCISION
C = CAUTERY
CR = CRYO
CU = CURETTAGE
O = OTHER

Appendix B   Computer record on database

OP RECORD

ID: [   ]   PT NUMBER: [   ]

SURNAME: [   ]

FIRST NAMES: [   ]

ADDRESS 1: [   ]

ADDRESS 2: [   ]

ADDRESS 3: [   ]

CITY: [   ]   POST CODE: [   ]

TEL NO: [   ]

DATE OF SURGERY: [   ]   FU DATE: [   ]

WRITTEN CONSENT: ☐   POST-OP WRITTEN INSTR: ☐

PRE-OP HISTO DIAGNOSIS: [   ]

PROCEDURE CODE: [   ]   SURGEON: [   ]

OP NOTES: [   ]

POST-OP HISTOLOGY: [   ]

POST-OP COMPLICATIONS: ☐   ADEQUACY OF EXCISION: ☐

INFLAMED WOUND: ☐   HAEMATOMA: ☐

WOUND BREAKDOWN: ☐   HAEMORRHAGE: ☐

WOUND INFECTION: ☐   STRETCHED SCAR: ☐

ABSCESS/DISCHARGE: ☐   KELOID: ☐

NOTES: [   ]

5

Local anaesthesia and nerve blocks

What higher aim can man attain than conquest over human pain?

Overview

- Methods of anaesthesia used in primary care.
- Types of local anaesthetics.
- Contraindications for LA.
- Methods of reducing pain of LA.
- Symptoms and signs of toxicity.
- Management of anaphylactic reaction.
- Use of adrenaline, including contraindications.
- Peripheral nerve blocks.
- Topical anaesthetics.

Introduction

The nature of primary-care surgery is such that almost all procedures are usually done by some form of local anaesthesia. However, depending on the experience of the 'anaesthetist', if appropriate equipment is available there is no reason for not being able to do procedures under regional or general anaesthesia.

Methods

The main methods of local anaesthesia used for minor surgery are mainly:

- infiltration anaesthesia
- peripheral nerve blocks
- topical anaesthesia (mucous membranes/skin).

Infiltration anaesthesia

Pain is a more terrible lord of mankind than even death himself.
Albert Schweitzer (1875–1965)

Infiltration anaesthesia is the injection of local anaesthetic agents into the dermis or deeper planes. Local anaesthetics are weak bases with a pH of just over 7.37. Chemically two types of local anaesthetic are available.

- Esters, e.g.:
  - cocaine (of historical interest) – cocaine spray has been found to be useful for topical spraying of oral or oropharyngeal regions
  - amethocaine, used for topical anaesthesia of skin and eye.

  Higher risk of allergic reactions; metabolised in tissue plasma.
- Amides. The three commonly used agents are:
  - lignocaine
  - bupivacaine
  - prilocaine.

  Safer, low risk of allergy; metabolised in the liver (caution in liver failure).

The drugs vary in their speed of onset, duration of action, potency, toxicity, stability, solubility and ability to penetrate mucous membranes, depending on drug factors and patient factors.

Drug factors

- Nature of drug
  - lignocaine, quick in onset
  - bupivacaine, slow
  - prilocaine, average.
- Strength and volume (dosage).

Patient factors

- Patient's age, weight and build.
- Site of injection: intradermal/intravascular/perineural. Inadvertent intravascular injection could lead to systemic toxicity. Avoid injecting into infected or inflamed tissue.
- Two important factors are local vascularity and amount of body fat.

How do local anaesthetics act?

- They prevent depolarisation and thereby inhibit conduction in a *reversible* way.
- Sensory fibres are blocked *faster* than motor fibres.
- Smaller-diameter pain fibres are blocked *before* the larger-diameter touch fibres.
- All local anaesthetics except cocaine cause vasodilatation.

Maximum dose of local anaesthetics

Lignocaine hydrochloride (plain)

Maximum dose for adult is 200 mg (if combined with adrenaline, the safe dosage goes up to 500 mg).

Strength (%)	Maximum volume (ml)
0.5	40
1	20
2	10
4	05

For the purpose of minor surgery, 1% plain lignocaine is the most commonly used strength.

Injection: 1% lignocaine hydrochloride (10 mg/ml) is available in 2 ml, 5 ml, 10 ml and 20 ml ampoules.

Remember

1 ml of 1% solution has 10 mg

Bupivacaine hydrochloride

Slow onset of action, takes nearly 30 minutes. Longer duration of action, about 8 hours in nerve blocks. Usual strength used is 0.25% (2.5 mg/ml), 10 ml ampoules.

Prilocaine hydrochloride

High doses can cause methaemoglobinaemia. The latter could be treated with intravenous methylene blue. Maximum dose for an adult is 400 mg when used alone.

Strengths are similar to those for lignocaine. But the 1% strength comes in only multi-dose vials. For minor-surgery settings, single-dose vials are more appropriate, reducing the chances of contamination. Useful for intravenous regional anaesthesia.

Recommended maximum doses with and without adrenaline

Drug	With adrenaline	Without adrenaline
Lignocaine	7 mg/kg body weight	3 mg/kg body weight
Bupivacaine	2 mg/kg body weight	2 mg/kg body weight
Prilocaine	9 mg/kg body weight	6 mg/kg body weight

Contraindications

- Known allergy to local anaesthetics. This is the only absolute contra-indication.
- Complete heart block.
- Hypovolaemia.
- Precaution in: severe associated illness; uncontrolled diabetes/ organ failure – cardiac/renal/liver (better referred to hospital due to increased risk).
- Caution in patients on anticoagulants.

Methods of reducing the pain of injection

- Always explain to the patient what you are going to do. Talking to the patient, and more importantly making the patient talk to you, helps to distract the patient and seems to have an analgesic effect! Vocal anaesthesia is important!
- If the patient has a quiet personality, making them bring saliva into their mouth while injecting may reduce the pain. A Spanish surgeon described this technique on a TV programme! Try it. This is rather 'soft' for the evidence-based diehards.
- Ensure that the solution is at body temperature. Solutions that are too cold can cause discomfort.[1] However, in another study[2] warming buffered lidocaine (lignocaine) did not reduce the pain of subcutaneous infiltration.
- Alkalinising the lignocaine, by mixing with sodium bicarbonate solution, helps to reduce the stinging/burning discomfort felt at the time of injection.[3,4]
- Using a topical anaesthetic prior to injection also reduces the discomfort. This is useful in younger, anxious patients.
- The finer the needle used, the lesser the pain felt. If large volumes have to be injected, or if the needle has to be manipulated in different directions, raise a small bleb of the anaesthetic before proceeding.
- Inject slowly.
- If long distances from the initial site of injection need to be covered, ensure that you proceed from an already anaesthetised area of skin.
- Give time for the anaesthetic to act! Test whether it is working before you start.
- Hypnotherapy and/or acupuncture are also used by some.

- When suturing a laceration, injecting the local anaesthetic from within the laceration is less painful than injecting via intact skin.[5]
- Gentleness in technique and a relaxed patient and doctor are perhaps the most important factors.

Symptoms and signs of toxicity

Systemic toxicity is usually due to large dose and/or vascularity of the injection site.

- CNS – confusion, convulsion, respiratory arrest.
- CVS – hypotension, bradycardia, cardiac arrest.
- Allergy/anaphylaxis – angio-oedema, urticaria, respiratory arrest.

Early

- Metallic taste
- Tinnitus
- Circum-oral numbness

Severe

- Slurred speech
- Jerky movements
- Tremor
- Hallucinations

Very severe

- Seizure
- Coma
- Respiratory depression
- Hypotension
- Bradycardia
- Asystole

Remember the early evidence of systemic toxicity

Management of anaphylactic reaction[6]

Initial therapy

1   *Secure and maintain airway: give 100% oxygen if possible.*
2   Lay patient flat with feet elevated, unless wheeze is the only symptom.
3   Intramuscular adrenaline (0.5–1 ml of 1 : 1000 for an adult). Repeat after 10 minutes until arterial pressure and pulse improves.
4   Set up an intravenous drip as soon as possible and give crystalloid or colloid, especially if there is hypotension.

Secondary therapy

1   Chlorpheniramine, slow intravenously (10 mg).
2   Intravenous hydrocortisone (100–300 mg).
3   Nebulised salbutamol for bronchospasm.
4   Aminophylline, slow intravenously (250 mg).
5   Observe for at least 2 hours after the acute episode. The patient should not be left alone for 24 hours after the attack. It is therefore better to admit the patient via 999.

Remember

All resuscitation equipment and drugs should not only be available but accessible quickly. They must be checked periodically for function, battery and expiry dates (drugs).

Use of adrenaline with local anaesthetic

•   Reduces absorption of local anaesthetic into the systemic circulation.
•   Reduces blood flow.
•   Reduces bleeding.
•   Increases duration of block.

Adrenaline is usually combined with lignocaine in a strength of 1 : 200 000 (5 μg/ml).

Contraindications to adrenaline

- Digits – fingers and toes
- Nose
- Ears
- Penis
- Peripheral vascular disease
- Past history of allergic reaction to adrenaline.

Reflections

When using combined preparations such as lignocaine + adrenaline, think twice!

Needles and syringes

- NHS needles are colour coded at the mount, from the finest 25 gauge, 17 mm length orange needle, through blue and green to white (Figure 5.1).
- The dental syringe needle is very fine, being 30 gauge and 30 mm long and double sided.
- NHS syringes are single-use, disposable, sterile syringes, available in 1 ml, 2 ml, 5 ml, 10 ml and 20 ml sizes.
- Dental syringes are made of metal and need to be purchased.

Remember

Always 'pull' before you 'push'.

Aspiration before injection helps you to avoid intravascular injection.

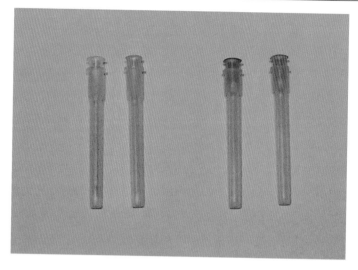

Figure 5.1 Commonly used needles.

Peripheral nerve blocks

- Used to anaesthetise the entire area supplied by a cutaneous nerve.
- The local anaesthetic is injected around the nerve and **never into** the nerve.
- May need higher concentration for thicker nerves.
- If injected into the nerve, invokes pain in the distribution of the nerve. The needle should ideally be withdrawn and the injection re-sited around the nerve.
- Used to anaesthetise a septic/inflamed area, by injecting the cutaneous nerves supplying the area, proximal to the site.

Commonly used peripheral nerve blocks

- Upper limb:
  - digital nerve block/ring block to fingers
  - median nerve block
  - ulnar nerve block
  - radial nerve block.
- Lower limb:
  - toe 'ring' block (for IGTN surgery)
  - posterior tibial nerve block (for procedures on the sole of the foot).

Remember

- **Never** inject into a nerve.
- Give adequate time for the anaesthetic to take effect.

Topical anaesthesia

Skin

Topical anaesthesia is useful for providing surface analgesia but it does not penetrate beyond the dermis. Useful for venepuncture and for cutaneous surgery in children and anxious adults with needle phobia. Topical anaesthesia is also useful for providing analgesia prior to epilation or treating telangiectasia with radiosurgery.

Emla® cream

Five per cent w/v; Astra. Available as 5 g tubes, which are useful for primary care (Figure 5.2). Emla is an acronym for eutectic mixture of amide group of local anaesthetics. The cream contains equal parts of lignocaine and prilocaine (lignocaine 25 mg and prilocaine 25 mg per gram of cream). It needs to be stored below 30°C. Shelf-life is about 3 years.

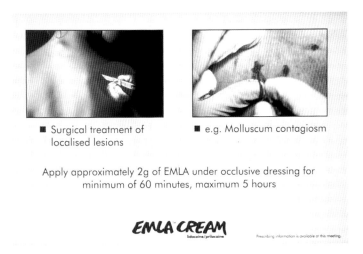

■ Surgical treatment of localised lesions

■ e.g. Molluscum contagiosm

Apply approximately 2g of EMLA under occlusive dressing for minimum of 60 minutes, maximum 5 hours

EMLA CREAM
lidocaine/prilocaine

Prescribing information is available at this meeting.

Figure 5.2 Emla® cream for use in minor surgery.

Advantage: refrigeration is not required if temperature is less than 30°C. There are three presentations. The 5 g tube is the most appropriate for primary care and each tube can be used twice. Emla® can be used for adults and children older than 1 year (compare with amethocaine). The contact time should be at least 1 hour before the procedure, and the cream should be covered by an occlusive dressing. Thicker skin may need a longer contact time. Effects last for up to 5 hours.

Special precautions: avoid applying to wounds, mucous membranes, or to patients with atopic eczema. It can cause transient local reactions of the skin.

Ametop® gel

Amethocaine 4% w/w gel; Smith & Nephew. Available as 1.5 g tubes. Can be bought over the counter. Needs to be stored below 15°C, and therefore *needs refrigeration* if stored for long periods. Amethocaine is an ester. The possibility of sensitisation from repeated exposure is not important in the context of primary-care surgery. Can be used for adults and children older than 1 month. The contact time is only about 30–45 minutes, before it becomes effective.

Emla® and amethocaine are available on the drug tariff and therefore prescribable. Their effectiveness diminishes rather quickly once the anaesthetic is wiped off from the skin prior to a procedure. They should *not* be used on open wounds, broken skin, lips, mouth or tongue, eyes, anal or genital regions.

ENT

Ten per cent lignocaine aerosol spray has been used to cause oropharyngeal anaesthesia. A ribbon containing 2% lignocaine and adrenaline can be used to anaesthetise the nose.

Eye

Amethocaine drops (0.5%) are used to anaesthetise the cornea and conjunctiva. It causes temporary stinging, but the onset of action is rapid and lasts for nearly an hour. The eye should be protected using an eye patch until the sensation returns. Useful for removal of foreign bodies from the cornea.

Reflections

- The latest editions of the *British National Formulary* and *MIMS* are worth reading.

- Be thorough with all aspects of the drugs you use in minor surgery.

References

1 Davidson JAH and Boom SJ. Warming lignocaine to reduce pain associated with injection. *BMJ*. 1992; **305**: 617–18.

2 Martin S, Jones JS and Wynn BN. Does warming local anesthetic reduce the pain of subcutaneous injection? *Am J Emerg Med*. 1996; **14**(1): 10–12.

3 Matsumoto AH, Reifsnyder AC, Hartwell GD *et al*. Reducing the discomfort of lidocaine administration through pH buffering. *J Vasc Interven Radiol*. 1994; **5**(1): 171–5.

4 Bartfield JM, Gennis P, Barbera J *et al*. Buffered versus plain lidocaine as a local anesthetic for simple laceration repair. *Ann Emerg Med*. 1990; **19**(12): 1387–9.

5 Bartfield JM, Sokaris SJ and Raccio-Robak N. Local anesthesia for lacerations: pain of infiltration inside vs outside the wound. *Acad Emerg Med*. 1998; **5**(2): 100–4.

6 Frew A. Anaphylaxis: a general practice guide to safe and effective treatment. *Pulse*. 1996; **25 May**: 86–7.

Further reading

Astra Pharmaceuticals. *Compendium of Regional Anaesthesia*. Undated.

This is an excellent short booklet of about 40 pages dealing with nerve blocks.

British National Formulary, No. 36, Chapter 15.2. British Medical Association and the Royal Pharmaceutical Society of Great Britain; 1998.

This gives a succinct account of the use, administration and toxicity of local anaesthetics and the use of vasoconstrictors. Lignocaine, bupivacaine, prilocaine, Ametop® and Emla® preparations are covered.

Eriksson E (ed.) *Illustrated Handbook of Local Anaesthesia* (2e). London, Lloyd-Luke (Medical Books) Ltd; 1979.

An excellent and comprehensive, but compact, book on local anaesthesia.

6

Common cutaneous lesions: benign lesions

The skin is the greatest barrier against the bug, and the best dressing

This chapter deals with the anatomy of the normal skin (Figure 6.1) and the more common benign lesions seen in primary care.

Overview

- Anatomy of the skin.
- Functions of the skin.
- Skin phototypes.
- Assessing skin lesions.
- Types of skin lesions:
  - benign
  - pre-malignant
  - malignant.
- Working diagnosis of skin lesions:
  - definitely benign
  - probably benign
  - probably malignant
  - definitely malignant.
- Benign cutaneous lesions: diagnosis and management.

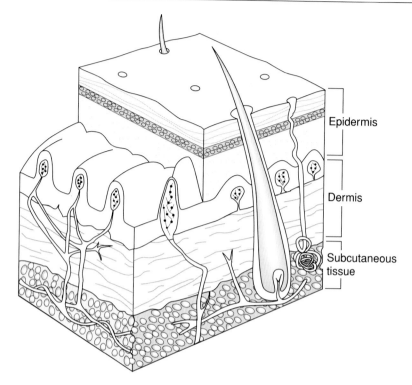

Figure 6.1 Anatomy of the normal skin.

Anatomy of the skin

Figure 6.1 illustrates the anatomy of the normal skin. The layers of the normal skin are:

- epidermis
- dermis
- subcuticular layer.

Epidermis

Comprises:

- stratum corneum, horny layer
- stratum lucidum, lucid layer (only palms and soles)
- stratum granularis, granular layer
- stratum spinosum, prickle layer
- stratum basalis, basal layer

superficial

↓

deep

The four types of cells in the epidermis are keratinocytes (85%), melanocytes, Langerhans cells and Merkel cells. The epidermis varies in thickness, depending on the area. It is about 0.05 mm thick. The dermis is about ten times thicker, being around 0.5 mm. Langerhans cells are analogous to macrophages and may play a role in immunity. Merkel cells are touch receptor cells present in the undersurface of the epidermis.

The horny layer is composed of stratified layers of dead keratin cells and keratin. Keratin is capable of absorbing vast amounts of water. The basal layer is a single layer of almost columnar cells. Keratinocytes and melanocytes are in this layer. Varying levels of differentiation of the keratinocytes are responsible for the histological differences in the appearance of the prickle layer, granular layer and lucid layer.

Dermis

Comprises:

- papillary dermis
- reticular dermis

↓ superficial
  deep

The dermis is composed of cells, fibres and amorphous ground substance. The main cells are fibroblasts. Other cells include mononuclear phagocytes, lymphocytes, Langerhans cells and mast cells. The fibres are mainly collagen bundles and, to a lesser extent, elastin fibres and reticulin fibres. The epidermis is interlocked to the dermis by the rete pegs from the lower surface of the epidermis, interlocking with the papillary ridges of the superior surface of the dermis (Figure 6.2).

Subcuticular layer (hypodermis/subcutaneous fat)

This layer of varying thickness is mainly adipose tissue and fibrous tissue. It supports the epidermis and the nerves and vessels traversing it to the skin. Fat is formed and stored in this layer. This allows for the mobility of skin. Skin incisions must extend vertically to this layer, when excising cutaneous lesions.

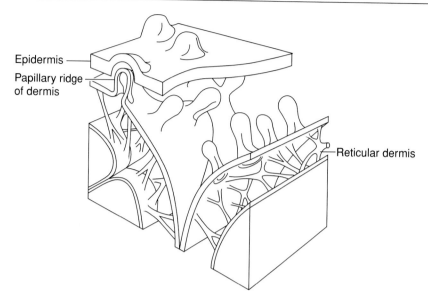

Epidermis

Papillary ridge
of dermis

Reticular dermis

Figure 6.2 Papillary ridges interlocking with undersurface of epidermis.

Epidermal appendages

The epidermal appendages are classified as *cornified* or *glandular*. The two cornified appendages are:

- nails
- hair.

The glandular appendages are:

- Sweat glands: eccrine and apocrine glands. Found universally in human skin. Most abundant in the axillae, palms and soles. (Now you know why some patients get cold, clammy hands!) Eccrine glands are small glands opening directly onto the skin surface. These glands are abundant in the palms and axillae and serve to maintain the internal body temperature. The apocrine are the larger glands that open into a hair follicle. The apocrine glands develop around puberty and are mainly located in the axillae and groin.
- Sebaceous glands (found in the obtuse angle of the hair follicle).

Apart from the nails, the appendages lie in the dermis. Remember that the sebaceous glands are absent in the palm and soles.

Functions of the skin

The five main functions of the skin are:

- protection: acts as the primary barrier against micro-organisms, gases, water; also prevents loss of fluids and body heat
- excretion of sweat
- sensation: the dermal papillae contain sensory nerve endings for touch, pressure, temperature and pain
- temperature regulation: via the dermal capillary circulation and the activity of the sweat glands
- synthesis of vitamin D with the help of ultraviolet light from the sun.

Most lesions removed by general practitioners are cutaneous or subcutaneous. Some of the more common lesions are on page 85. The list is by no means comprehensive.

Skin phototypes

There are three skin colours for practical purposes: white (Caucasian), brown (e.g. Asian) and black (e.g. African).

There are six skin phototypes (based on colour, sun-burning and tanning properties):

- type 1: white skin that burns easily and does not tan

- type 2: white skin that burns easily and tans with difficulty

- type 3: white skin that burns rarely and tans easily

- type 4: white skin that does not burn, and tans easily

- type 5: brown skin

- type 6: black skin

The single question to ask a patient is: 'Do you tan easily?'
If the answer is no, the patient is either type 1 or 2, both being at higher risk for melanoma.

Assessing skin lesions

When assessing these lesions, two important questions to ask are:

- *Where is it?*, i.e. anatomical site and plane of origin of the lesion
- *What is it?*, i.e. what is the nature of the lesion?

Can you make a pathological diagnosis, clinically? This is a very useful exercise, and by following up the histology of the lesion, you could enhance your diagnostic accuracy of these lesions. However, the final diagnosis of the nature and pathology of any lesion is histological. Therefore checking the pathologist's report is mandatory. It is good practice to send all lesions that are excised for histological examination. However, with increasing experience, you will note that it will not be cost-effective to send some obvious lesions, such as small skin tags and viral warts, for histology. The pathologist needs good clinical information to give a good histological report. If you wish to be cautious, offer the specimen (in a fixative) for the patient to keep (!) or ask the patient his/her preference. Document the outcome of your counselling if the specimen is not sent for histology. Familiarise yourself by looking at patients in a dermatology clinic, or observing all the cutaneous lesions you see when examining patients for whatever reason. Looking at good dermatology atlases periodically and attempting to diagnose the lesions before reading the text helps to improve your diagnostic skills.

In the management of cutaneous lesions, other questions that arise are:

- What are the options for management? What are their pros and cons?
- What would happen if you did nothing?
- Which option will you choose and why?
- When will you treat?
- How will you treat it?

Have you ensured that the patient understands what you plan to do, and makes an informed choice?

All surgeons who operate on cutaneous lesions should be able to at least differentiate between benign and malignant lesions. Clinically the lesions could be classified into:

☺ definitely benign
☺ probably benign
☹ probably malignant
☹ definitely malignant.

It would be wise to refer those lesions that are definitely malignant on clinical examination, unless you are familiar with the definitive management of the lesion. Whether a probably malignant lesion should be referred, depends on your experience. Most general practitioners will manage the benign and probably benign lesions. Ensure that a complete excision is done with a normal margin of 2 mm for the probably benign or malignant lesions. A useful policy is: if in doubt, refer!

Benign lesions

Beauty is skin deep; and so are most cutaneous lesions!

Checklist of lesions

- warts
- skin tags (fibroepithelioma/acrochordons [Greek, *akros* = tip, *chorde* = string/cord])
- benign histiocytomas (dermatofibroma)
- seborrhoeic wart (basal cell papilloma)
- molluscum contagiosum (Latin, *mollis* = soft)
- keratoacanthoma (Greek, *keras, keratos* = horn: horny layer of skin; *akantha* = thorn) (molluscum sebaceum)
- freckles
- pyogenic granuloma
- blue naevus
- halo naevus
- Spitz naevus
- congenital melanocytic naevus
- benign melanocytic naevus: junctional, compound, intradermal
- dysplastic melanocytic naevi (DMN)/atypical mole syndrome
- De Morgan spots and other vascular angiomas
- spider naevi
- sebaceous cysts
- lipomas (subcutaneous and deeper planes).

Describing skin lesions

The morphology and distribution of skin lesions often indicate the diagnosis. It is useful to remember the common terminology used to describe skin lesions. Scratching, ulceration or secondary infection may modify the primary morphology of skin lesions. Try to identify the primary lesions and secondary lesions.

Primary lesions

> *The beginning of wisdom is the definition of terms.*
>
> Socrates (470–399 BC)

Depending on their size, five major types of primary lesions are described.

1 Flat, coloured lesions (flush with the skin): macule or patch lesions. Macular lesion: a macule (Latin, *macula* = a spot) is a coloured lesion of the skin *less than* 5 mm in size without any elevation or depression, i.e. it is not palpable though visible. A patch is more than 5 mm in diameter. The lesions may be hypo- or hyper-pigmented. If the colour is due to extravasation of blood, a different terminology is used (see below).

2 Elevated solid lesions could either be a papule, nodule or plaque. A papule (Latin, *paula* = a pimple) is a well circumscribed elevation above the skin (and hence palpable), less than 5 mm in diameter or elevation. A nodule (Latin, *nodulus* = a small knot) is more than 5 mm in size but less than 20 mm (2 cm). A plaque (French, *plaque* = plate) is more than 2 cm in diameter, but a 'thin' elevation. While a papule is mostly from epidermal cells or melanocytes, a nodule may arise from the epidermis, dermis or deeper subcutaneous tissue. Nodules may indicate systemic disease with cutaneous or subcutaneous manifestation (e.g. rheumatoid disease, tuberculosis, mycoses, lymphomas, metastatic disease, or from metabolic disorders such as gout). When assessing elevated lesions, try to assess the 'depth' of the lesion by trying to pick the lesion with the skin between the thumb and index finger. It also gives an idea of the plane of origin – whether the lesion is primarily in the skin or under the skin.

3 Fluid-filled lesions could either be a vesicle or bulla. A vesicle is less than 5 mm in diameter and a bulla is more than 5 mm in diameter.

4 Pus-filled lesions could be pustules or abscesses. A pustule is a circumscribed collection of pus (abscess) which is less than 5 mm in diameter. (In 'folliculitis' often small pustules may form as a complication.) When over 5 mm in diameter, it is known as an abscess.

5 Extravasation of blood into skin or fluid. Extravasation of blood leads to the following types of conditions:
   • petechiae (pin-head size)
   • purpura (less than 2 mm in diameter)
   • ecchymosis (over 2 mm in diameter).

Extravasation of fluid into the dermis leads to wheals with elevation of the skin. Wheals caused by trauma usually disappear within 72 hours. Urticarial wheals caused by allergy or vasculitis usually last longer. Angio-oedema is more extensive and also involves the subcutaneous tissue.

Secondary lesions

Secondary lesions include scales, crusts, keratoses, fissures, erosions, ulceration, atrophy and lichenification.

Warts and verrucae

There was a young lady named Rose
Who had a huge wart on her nose
When she had it removed
Her appearance improved
But her glasses slipped down to her toes.
Contributed by a course participant!

Warts are caused by the human papilloma virus (HPV), and found in the top layer of the skin. Viral warts/verrucae (warts in the foot) are the most common benign lesions for which patients consult their general practitioner. Of the more than 50 HPV types, the community viral warts are caused by about eight.[1] The common warts (verruca vulgaris) are caused by HPV1, HPV2, HPV4 and HPV7. A significant proportion of the referrals to a dermatologist (10–25%) is for viral warts. The majority of warts tend to disappear with time. In one study, about two-thirds of the lesions resolved spontaneously within 2 years.[2] The main reason for consultation is cosmetic. Some warts and verrucae are painful, especially those on the sole of the foot. With the ever-increasing financial constraints on the National Health Service, some would argue that warts and veruccae should not be treated on the NHS.[3] Explanation and conservative self-management plans should be attempted before treating by cautery or curettage or cryotherapy or excision.

Types of warts

Classified according to the site.

- Common hand warts (verruca vulgaris).

- Foot warts/plantar warts (verruca plantaris). When grouped together they are known as mosaic warts.
- Flat warts (verruca planaris). Less rough and usually found on the face in children. They tend to arise in the bearded area of adult males and on the legs of females, both probably related to shaving.
- Genital warts (condylomata acuminata).

The majority of the common warts occur in children over the age of 5 and in young adults. Genital warts, found in adults, are sexually transmitted and therefore need to be managed by a genito-urinary specialist, as contact tracing will be an important issue.

Hand warts are found on the peri-ungual skin or on the dorsum of the hand. Warts should not be confused with *corns* or *calluses*. Corns and calluses are produced by friction. Both are thickenings of the skins and do not have 'roots' like warts. Corns occur over small localised areas, often on the dorsum of the toes as a result of abnormal structure of the anatomy below and the shoes worn, e.g. from hammer toes or exostoses. They could also occur on the plantar surface of the foot, especially over the metatarsal heads. Calluses are more diffuse, over a larger area of skin, commonly on the plantar aspect of the foot. Corns, unlike warts, exhibit normal skin ridges over their surface. They do not bleed when pared. On paring viral warts one often sees 'blackheads'/punctate dark spots, from thrombosed microvessels, or active bleeding from 'feeder' vessels.

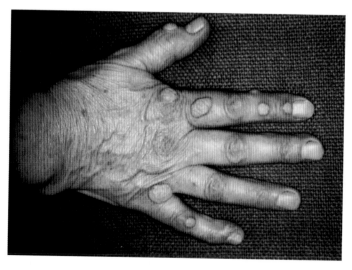

Figure 6.3 Viral warts on the hand (courtesy of Dr C Grattan).

Self-management/conservative treatment

Most warts in children will disappear with time. About two-thirds will resolve within 2 years. Advise children who have a tendency to nail-bite to stop doing so. But habits are difficult to change!

Genital warts can predispose to cancer. There is a higher risk of cancer of the cervix in females with genital warts. Peri-anal warts in young children should alert the general practitioner to the possibility of sexual abuse.

Medical/conservative treatment includes

Advice on the use of topical applications bought over the counter (OTC) from a chemist. This includes preparations containing varying strengths of salicylic acid with or without lactic acid. Using occlusive dressing to cover the wart after applying salicylic acid enhances the efficacy of this treatment.[4] Formaldehyde preparations are also available. The latter tends to stain the skin, but is useful for mosaic warts. They are all keratolytics, which help in the involution of the warts. But they need to be applied daily for at least 2–3 months, and this requires patience and perseverance. They are contraindicated for the face and genital warts. Some of the OTC and prescription preparations include: Bazuka® gel (salicylic acid, 12%; lactic acid, 4%), Cuplex® gel (salicylic acid, 11%; lactic acid, 4%), Duofilm® paint or Salactol® paint (salicylic acid, 16.7%; lactic acid, 16.7%), Occlusal® (salicylic acid, 26%), Salactac® gel (salicylic acid, 12%; lactic acid, 4%) and Verrugon® ointment (salicylic acid, 50%).

Larger warts need to be pared down before application of the paints or gels. An emery board or skin scraper could be used. It is worth rubbing these warts using a pumice stone when having a bath.

CIMETIDINE (TAGAMET®) THERAPY
Cimetidine, by enhancing the immune system, may have an effect in the involution of the wart. However, other H_2-receptor antagonists have not been shown to be as effective. The dosage for adults is 400 mg for 8 weeks, in addition to the use of salicylic acid, and in children 20–40 mg/kg/day in divided doses is recommended for 8 weeks. Unfortunately there are as yet no randomised control trials.

Other medical treatments

These include individual wart injection with bleomycin. This could be painful. Immunotherapy methods invoking an allergy by the patients to chemicals have been tried. Podophyllin preparations have been licensed for the treatment of genital warts. Hypnotherapy has also been utilised as a modality of treatment on patients with multiple warts.[5,6]

It is worth remembering the golden rule for any therapeutic intervention:

The remedy should not be worse than the malady!

Surgical treatments

These include (4Cs):

- cryotherapy
- cautery
- curettage or
- cutting out or excision of the lesion, by scalpel or radiosurgery.

The choice depends on the five 'A's described previously (age, associated illness, allergies, anxiety, anticoagulant treatment) *and* the site and number of warts needing treatment.

CRYOTHERAPY

If using Histofreezer, you will need to pare down the lesion before treating. Histofreezer is not good for large warts. Cryotherapy may usually require more than one treatment at weekly or fortnightly intervals. The aim is to raise a blister to destroy the wart and then allow healing to occur. Using a double freeze–thaw cycle may not be of any advantage over a single freeze–thaw cycle in the treatment of hand warts, but may be far more effective for plantar warts.[7]

CAUTERY

Cautery for larger, solitary warts can be performed under local anaesthetic. Chemical cautery using silver nitrate sticks has also been reported.[8] Electrocautery using a hyfrecator to fulgarate lesions is an alternative method. Radiosurgery could also be used to fulgarate lesions.

CURETTAGE

Under local anaesthetic large verrucae or warts could be curetted out, and healing allowed to occur by secondary intention. This takes time. Haemostasis could be achieved by coagulation using the hyfrecator or radiosurgery ball electrodes.

CUTTING OR EXCISION

Excision under local anaesthetic can be used for longstanding solitary warts. The wound could be sutured primarily, or allowed to heal by secondary intention.

Reflections

- Have you devised a written instruction in the form of a leaflet, for patients, on warts?

- How do you distinguish between warts and corns and calluses?

Skin tags (benign fibroepitheliomas or acrochordons)

These are usually very small and pedunculated lesions that increase in number with age. They are commonly found around the neck, axillae and upper trunk. The pedicles are usually about 2 mm or less in thickness. They are easily managed by cautery excision without an anaesthetic.

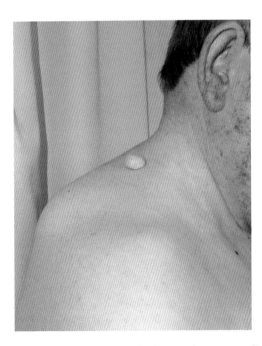

Figure 6.4 18 mm wide fibroepithelioma and a large subcutaneous lipoma causing a hump near the base of neck.

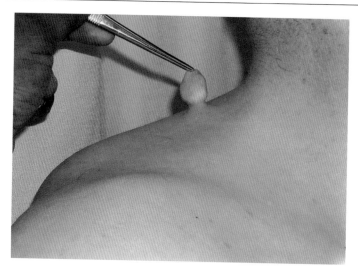

Figure 6.5 Fibroepithelioma lifted to show a wide pedicle.

Larger lesions, with sessile bases may need a local anaesthetic and even suturing if indicated. Cryotherapy and snipping with a sharp scissors can also be used. Radiosurgical excision is an alternative method. A circular or diamond-shaped loop electrode in cutting mode with power around 3, on an Ellman Surgitron FFPF will effectively excise the lesion. If performed under local anaesthetic, the base could be planed flush with the skin.

Dermatofibroma (benign histiocytoma)

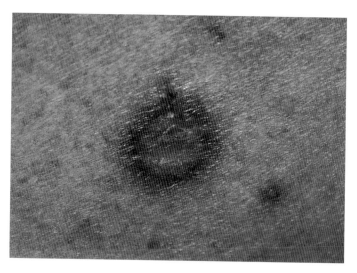

Figure 6.6 Dermatofibroma (courtesy of Dr C Grattan).

Common. Presents as a firm or hard, itchy nodule of the skin, sometimes after an insect bite. Characteristically causes 'dimpling' when squeezed between two fingers (Fitzpatrick's sign), or if the skin is stretched on either side of the lesion. This is *not* pathognomonic of dermatofibroma.[9] If you decide to treat, a shave biopsy with a blade or with radiosurgery is effective. Depending on the site, excision biopsy could be done under local anaesthesia.

Seborrhoeic wart (basal cell papilloma)

The classical lesion is *greasy* and looks as if it is *stuck on* the skin. In older patients it is more crumbly and less greasy looking. Cryotherapy, shave biopsy, flush curettage, electrofulgaration, radiosurgical shaving or excision are the various options of treatment, if the patient wishes it removed. If the lesion is pigmented and if you are not definite of the diagnosis, it is safer **not** to use cryotherapy, as you cannot biopsy the lesion, and you may be dealing with a nodular melanoma. However the latter *usually* exhibits colour variability. If in doubt, either refer the patient, or completely excise the lesion with at least 2 mm normal margin and send for urgent histology. The patient must be followed up. You should have a practice protocol (with separate operation book/computerised record) for the histological follow-up of lesions (*see* Chapter 3).

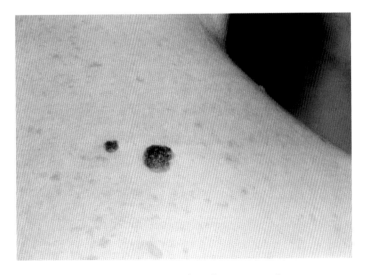

Figure 6.7 Seborrhoeic keratosis (courtesy of Professor R Mackie).

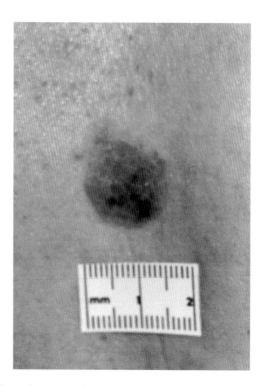

Figure 6.8 Seborrhoeic keratosis showing 'greasy' surface (courtesy of Professor R Mackie).

Molluscum contagiosum

Umbilicated papular lesions caused by a pox virus. Usually multiple, and found in children and young adults. More common in patients with atopic eczema. Best left alone since the majority resolve in a few months. Patients and parents need to be counselled on natural history. Could be pricked with cautery, desiccated, curetted under topical anaesthesia or treated with focused cryotherapy. The latter could cause scarring and hyperpigmentation.

Keratoacanthoma (molluscum sebaceum)

Fast-growing lesions, usually on sun-exposed skin of elderly patients. History is often of a lesion of a few weeks. More common in the head.

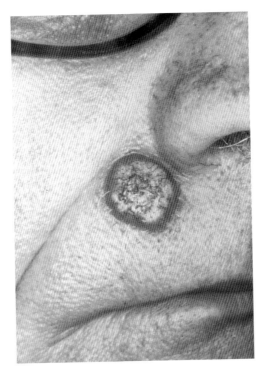

Figure 6.9 Keratoacanthoma (courtesy of Professor R Mackie).

The short history and central crater of a keratin plug is characteristic. They resolve spontaneously over the next few months, **but** rarely the base may be a squamous cell carcinoma. Always examine the base carefully, under magnification if necessary. If you have doubts, refer the patient or excise the lesion completely and send for histology, before any definitive action. If you choose to do nothing, you must monitor the patient periodically over the next few months until the lesion disappears. Follow-up is vital, as the small potential for an early squamous cell carcinoma at the base has to be excluded.

Freckles (ephelides)

Usually found in sun-exposed areas. Light tan or brown macules, more common in adolescents and young adults, though it can occur at any age. More common in blonde or red-haired people. Darken further on sun

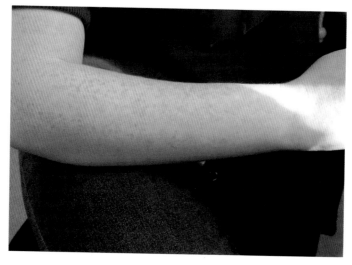

Figure 6.10 Freckles on forearm of adolescent girl.

exposure. Increased melanin is seen in the basal layer of the epidermis, *without* an increase in the number of melanocytes. Lentigo (or lentigines), on the other hand, exhibit an increase in the total number of melanocytes. Significance: it is an *independent risk factor* for the development of malignant melanomas. No treatment is required. But advise on sun protection (sun screen, avoiding midday sun, appropriate clothing and hats).

Pyogenic granuloma

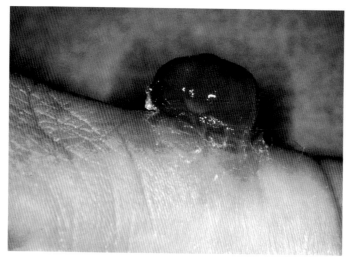

Figure 6.11 Pyogenic granuloma on finger (courtesy of Dr C Grattan).

Rapidly developing haemangiomatous lesion, after minor trauma or sepsis. They are solitary vascular nodules that bleed easily. Cannot exclude an amelanotic melanoma. Therefore, whatever method of treatment used, histology of the lesion is mandatory.

Benign melanocytic lesions

Blue naevus

The blue-black colour is due to the pigment cells being deep in the dermis. The colour is uniformly dark, not variegated. They are symmetrical with well-defined borders, and dome shaped. More common in teens or young adulthood. They are permanent. Not necessary to remove, unless for cosmetic reasons.

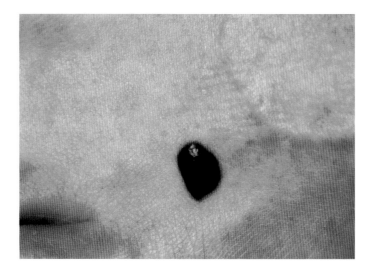

Figure 6.12 Blue naevus (courtesy of Dr C Grattan).

Halo naevus

Seen in the trunk of teenagers, during summer months. The halo of depigmentation is due to the absence of melanin. When left alone, the central naevus usually disappears. The halo regains its pigmentation, which may take from months to years.

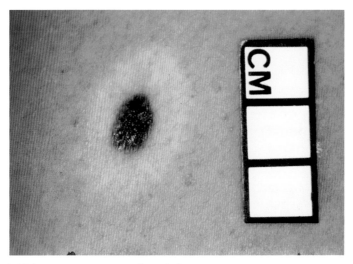

Figure 6.13 Halo naevus (courtesy of Dr C Grattan).

Spitz naevus*

Commonly seen on the face of adolescent children. Red cherry-like domed lesions, which can grow rapidly over a few months. They are benign and uncommon.

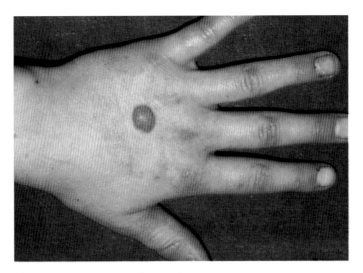

Figure 6.14 Spitz naevus (courtesy of Dr C Grattan).

*S Spitz, US pathologist. Born 1910

Congenital melanocytic naevus

Usually hairy, occur in about 1% of newborns. They tend to grow larger with the child. Large naevi need referral to a plastic surgeon.

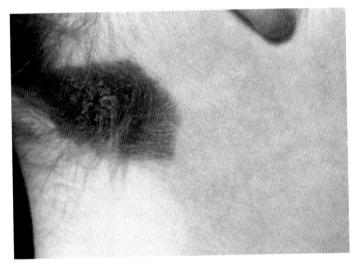

Figure 6.15 Congenital naevus (courtesy of Professor R Mackie).

Benign melanocytic naevus: junctional, compound or intradermal

These are all *acquired* naevi. Depending on the different stages of maturation of the naevus, the three types are found at different ages. The junctional naevus is found in children and adolescents, and is usually a macular lesion. The compound naevus occurs in young adults, and the intradermal naevus in older adults. They are both maculo-papular, raised above the surface of the skin. The former is usually pigmented. Compound naevi are usually domed and mamillated at the centre, especially when magnified or examined with a dermatoscope.

Dysplastic melanocytic naevus (DMN)

Also known as atypical melanocytic naevus or atypical mole syndrome (AMS) or dysplastic melanocytic syndrome (familial).

*   May occur singly or in multiples.
*   Sporadic or familial (autosomal dominant).

- Difficult to differentiate from early superficial spreading malignant melanoma/lentigo maligna/pigmented intradermal naevus/compound naevus.

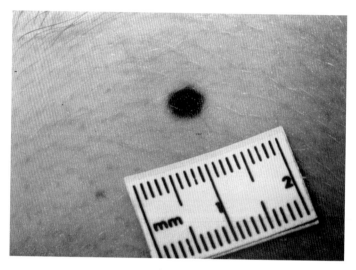

Figure 6.16 Benign compound naevus (courtesy of Professor R Mackie).

CLINICAL CHARACTERISTICS AND IMPORTANT POINTS TO CONSIDER

- Usually larger than the benign moles. Usually 2–10 mm.
- Can occur at any age, in both males and females.
- May be asymmetrical in shape.
- Border usually *not* well defined, may appear inflamed and *fuzzy*.
- Colour may *not* be uniform.
- Surface is usually smooth (macular).
- Always look for multiple moles and count them, both on the trunk and lower limbs.
- Multiple freckles are an independent risk factor for malignant melanoma.
- Always ask for a family history of dysplastic moles or malignant melanoma.
- Always ask for a past history of malignant melanoma.

MANAGEMENT

Each DMN must be assessed individually and collectively in the context of the previous and family history. They are best excised with a margin of 1–2 mm and sent for histology.

> ### Remember
>
> - The greater the number of dysplastic naevi, the greater the risk of malignant melanoma.
>
> - The majority of malignant melanomas arise spontaneously, rather than from a pre-existing dysplastic naevus.
>
> - Examination under magnification is useful in determining the nature of the lesion.
>
> - Changes in *size*, *shape* and *colour* constitute the three major signs of malignant melanoma.
>
> - **All melanocytic naevi** or **any pigmented lesion** should be sent for histology. It would be medico-legally **negligent** not to do so.

The naevi count in children living closer to the equator is more than in those who are away from it. A comparison of the naevi of school-children in Australia and Scotland by Fritschi *et al.*[10] showed that the children in Brisbane had significantly more naevi than the children in Glasgow. Other significant predictive factors include freckles and skin type. The *risk* of malignant melanoma was higher when there were *four or more atypical naevi*; or *100 or more benign naevi* of more than 2 mm diameter.[11] Red hair has a protective effect!

Risk factors for developing malignant melanoma

☹ Skin that burns easily, rather than tans. Previous history of recurrent sunburn.

☹ Family history of DMN (dysplastic naevus syndrome).

☹ Family history of malignant melanoma.

☹ Past history of malignant melanoma.

☹ Blonde hair.

☹ Blue eyes.

☹ Multiple freckles/lentigines.

☹ Multiple dysplastic naevi (>100 benign naevi or >3 atypical naevi).

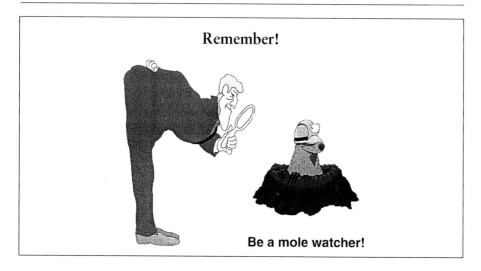

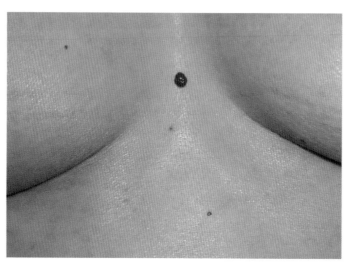

Figure 6.17 De Morgan cherry angioma of chest.

De Morgan spots* (cherry angiomata) and other vascular angiomas

Characteristics:

- age: usually above 40 years; depends on duration of sun exposure
- sex: males and females
- site: usually trunk
- size: 2–5 mm usually

*Campbell De Morgan, British physician (1811–1876)

- symmetry: symmetrical
- surface: papular
- border: well defined
- colour: cherry red/angiomatous.

These are harmless, and best left alone.

Spider naevi (spider telangiectasias)

These are not tumours. They are telangiectasias, which are 0.1–1 mm wide venules, capillaries or arterioles. Reddish and Pelzer[12] classified telangiectasias into four types (Figure 6.18):

- simple (linear)
- arborised
- spider (star)
- papular (puntiform).

Characteristics:

- age: usually in adults over 40
- sex: possibly more common in females; more females seek help
- site: anywhere; more common in head, trunk and lower limbs

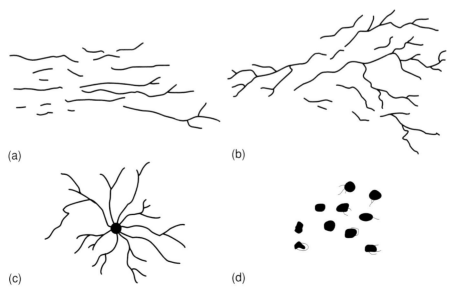

(a)

(b)

(c)

(d)

Figure 6.18 Four types of telangiectasia: (a) Linear telangiectasia; (b) Arborising telangiectasia; (c) Spider naevi; (d) Papular telangiectasia.

- size: varies; central vessel with radiating linear vessels; feeding vessel arteriole in upper half of the body
- symmetry: usually symmetrical (spider naevi)
- surface: mainly macular (arteriolar spider naevi); venular spider naevi are elevated
- border: well defined
- colour: those developing from the arteriolar end of the capillary loop tend to be more red and macular; those arising from the venular end are bluish and protrude above the surface of the skin. Pressure on the central vessel causes blanching and disappearance of radiating vessels.

Sebaceous cysts (epidermoid cysts/pilar cysts)

If you want to converse with me, define your terms.

Voltaire (1694–1778)

Semantics

The true sebaceous cyst in histopathological terms is relatively rare, containing oily sebum. The true sebaceous cyst in histological terms is known as steatocytoma multiplex. It arises from a failure of canalisation between the sebaceous lobules and the follicular pore.

The usual sebaceous cyst known to physicians and surgeons is lined by a keratin wall and contains smelly, greasy contents with the consistency of toothpaste. These keratinous cysts (sebaceous cysts) are of two types:

1 epidermoid cysts (keratin wall similar to epidermis), situated anywhere except the scalp
2 trichilemmal cysts (lined by cells resembling the external root sheath of a hair follicle). The classical site is those arising from the scalp. Their walls are thicker, and easier to dissect and 'deliver' like a baby's head, *in toto*, giving a special obstetric thrill.[13] They are familial.[14]

Epidermoid cysts

Characteristics:

- age: any age, usually adults
- sex: either
- site: face, neck, upper trunk (sites common for acne)
- size: usually <2 cm

- symmetry: symmetrical, dome-shaped lump attached to the skin
- surface: smooth, punctum with keratin plug may be present
- border: smooth edge, mobile – especially 'virgin' cysts, i.e. no previous episodes of infection
- colour: usually same as skin; cysts very close to the surface and stretching the skin, as in the ear lobes, are more whitish or yellow in colour.

Trichilemmal cysts (pilar cysts)

Same as above, except that they are located in the scalp. Easier to dissect and 'deliver', without puncturing the cyst wall.

Complications

- Increase in size, with pressure to adjoining structures and discomfort.
- Sepsis with abscess formation; painful.

Management

Excison under local anaesthetic. If an abscess forms, it needs incision and drainage, followed by antibiotics, packing and dressing. A definitive excision could be done after the inflammation settles. In the early stages of abscess formation with cellulitis, I start on a course of flucloxacillin (if the patient is not allergic to penicillin). About 48 hours later, when the inflammation is more circumscribed, rather than diffused, and the abscess localised, the incision and drainage can be done effectively. It is worth attempting to dissect and excise the wall of the cavity, as it is easier to find the tissue planes after a few days of antibiotics. However, if the patient presents with severe pain from an abscess, drainage should not be delayed.

Excision is usually done under local anaesthetic. Various incisions have been used. They are either linear incisions of varying lengths (Figure 6.19) or ellipses (Figure 6.20) to include the punctum. Of the linear incisions shown in Figure 6.19, (a) leaves a long scar; (b) can identify the edge of the cyst and dissect from the edge, leaving a smaller scar; and (c) involves minimal incision,[15] followed by opening and emptying cyst, and then dissecting the wall out; the wound is sutured, leaving a smaller scar. This

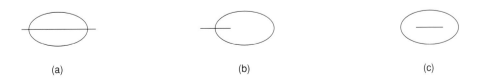

(a) (b) (c)

Figure 6.19 Excision of sebaceous cyst: linear incisions.

(a)   (b)

Figure 6.20 Excision of sebaceous cyst: elliptical incisions.

takes longer. An even smaller incision, microincision,[16] followed by expressing the contents, removing the cyst wall, and *not* closing the wound has been described.

Figure 6.20(a) shows a mainly linear incision, with a small ellipse to include the punctum. A modification of this is the use of a trephining technique[17] using a 3 mm biopsy punch under local anaesthetic, including the punctum, emptying the contents, and dissecting and removing the wall through the wound. The wound is initially packed and after 2 days allowed to heal on its own, without suturing. Figure 6.20(b) shows a wide ellipse. This is *not* necessary for sebaceous cysts, although it may be appropriate for small cutaneous lesions. There is too much normal skin excision, by sticking to the 3 : 1 rule to prevent dog-ears when suturing. I usually use a circular incision for small lesions of less than about 7 mm diameter.

Lipomas (subcutaneous and deeper planes) (*see* Figure 6.4)

Lipomas could be excised under local anaesthetic. Usually linear incision is used. The lipoma is dissected using small, curved, blunt-nosed scissors; and for deeper lipomas, by using larger scissors such as the Mayo dissecting scissors. Obliterate dead space, and ensure haemostasis before closure.

> ### Reflections
>
> • The skin is the largest organ of the human body and the armour protecting the body from the environment.
>
> • It is important to be able to make a clinical diagnosis of the common cutaneous lesions.
>
> *continued*

continued

- It is useful to be able to differentiate between a macule, patch, papule, nodule, pustule, vesicle and bulla.

- It is worth 'sitting in' with a consultant at the hospital, if he or she runs a 'see and treat' skin lesion clinic or mole clinic.

- It will be useful to look at some of the dermatology atlases, and do a self-assessment of your competence at diagnosing the cutaneous lesions from the photographs. Some of the books worth looking at are listed in Further reading. Alternatively, you could browse the textbooks in the dermatology section of your local medical library.

- Another useful exercise is to take a polaroid photograph, or a digital photograph, of lesions you see in your patients and discuss them with your local friendly dermatologist!

Some useful www sites

1   Dermatology atlas: this is an excellent site for reviewing your diagnostic skills by looking at images of good clarity:
    http://www.derma.med.uni-erlangen.de/index_e.htm
    The University of Erlangen in Germany provides the Dermatology Internet Service (DermIS) from which you can access the Dermatology Online Atlas.
2   Physicians' choice: gives access by links to almost all the useful websites for a family physician: *www.mdchoice.com/pcsites.htm*

Frequently asked questions

Q. What are the clinical features that help in the diagnosis of a sebaceous cyst?
A. A lump arising in the skin. The skin cannot be picked up separately from the lump. A punctum is almost pathognomonic. The lump is 'soft' in consistency.

Q. Is it mandatory to remove the entire cyst wall *in toto*?

A. It is good practice to attempt to remove the entire cyst with its content, *in toto* via *standard* incisions. It is not always easy to do so in epidermoid cysts. The principle is to attempt to remove the entire wall of the cyst. If the entire wall cannot be removed by dissection, especially in cysts which have been infected or inflamed in the past, it is worth curetting the cavity or using other means such as electrodessication or cautery. If you accidentally cut into the cyst, applying a curved artery forceps against the hole enables you to proceed with your dissection and excision.

Q. Why do some patients get recurring sebaceous cysts?

A. Some patients have a predisposition for multiple and/or recurrent sebaceous cysts. The recurrence at the same site is often attributed to incomplete removal of the cyst wall on the previous occasion. Often these are not true recurrences, but the development of new epidermoid cysts in the same area. It is worth excluding diabetes mellitus in patients who get multiple or recurrent sebaceous cysts, as we do for patients developing carbuncles.

Q. What is a 'virgin' sebaceous cyst?

A. It is a cyst that has never been inflamed or infected. These are easier to dissect.

References

1 Shah KV and Howley PM. Papillomaviruses. In: BN Fields, DM Knipe *et al.* (eds) *Virology* (2e). New York, Raven Press; 1990.

2 Massing AM and Epstein WL. Natural history of warts. A two-year study. *Arch Dermatol.* 1963; 87: 306–10.

3 Bridger PC and Banatvala JE. *Minor surgery in primary care – warts and all.* Bandolier Internet publication. *www.jr2.ox.ac.uk/bandolier/bandopubs/wart.html* 1996; *Bandolier* 31.

4 Veien NK, Madsen SM, Avrach W *et al.* The treatment of plantar warts with a keratolytic agent and occlusion. *J Dermatol Treat.* 1991; 2: 59–61.

5 Sinclair-Gieben AHC and Chalmers D. Evaluation of treatment of warts by hypnosis. *Lancet.* 1959; 7: 21–2.

6 Spanos NP, Williams V and Gwynn MI. Effects of hypnotic, placebo, and salicylic acid treatments on wart regression. *Psychosom Med.* 1990; 52: 109–14.

7   Berth-Jones J, Bourke J, Eglitis H *et al*. Value of second freeze-thaw cycle in cryotherapy of common warts. *Br J Dermatol*. 1994; **131**(6): 883–6.

8   Yazar S and Basaran E. Efficacy of silver nitrate pencils in the treatment of common warts. *J Dermatol*. 1994; **21**: 329–33.

9   Meffert JJ, Peake ME and Wilde JL. 'Dimpling' is not unique to dermato-fibromas. *Dermatology*. 1997; **195**(4): 384–6.

10   Fritschi L, McHenry P, Green A, Mackie R, Green L and Siskind V. Naevi in schoolchildren in Scotland and Australia. *Br J Dermatol*. 1994; **130**(5): 599–603.

11   Bataille V, Bishop JA, Sasieni P *et al*. Risk of cutaneous melanoma in relation to the numbers, types and sites of naevi: a case-control study. *Br J Cancer*. 1996; **73**(2): 1605–11.

12   Reddish W and Pelzer RH. Localised vascular dilatations of the human skin: Capillary microscopy and related studies. *Am Heart J*. 1949; **37**: 106.

13   Comaish S. Treatment of sebaceous cysts: Comment. *The Practitioner*. 1989; **233**: 700–1.

14   Leppard BJ, Sanderson KV and Wells RS. Hereditary trichilemmal cysts. Hereditary pilar cysts. *Clin Exp Dermatol*. 1977; **2**: 23–32.

15   Vivakananthan C. Minimal incision for removing sebaceous cysts. *Br J Plast Surg*. 1972; **25**: 60.

16   Avakoff JC. Microincision for removing sebaceous cysts. *Plast Reconst Surg*. 1989; **84**(1): 173–4.

17   Richards MA. Trephining large sebaceous cysts. *Br J Plast Surg*. 1985; **38**: 583–5.

Further reading

Fitzpatrick TB, Johnson RA, Wolff K, Polano MK and Suurmond D. *Colour Atlas and Synopsis of Clinical Dermatology* (3e). New York, McGraw Hill; 1997.

This book is worth having in the practice library. Also available on CD-Rom.

Hunter JAA, Savin JA and Dahl MV. *Clinical Dermatology* (2e). Oxford, Blackwell Science; 1995.

The chapter on diagnosis of skin disorders is very useful for general practitioners.

Lachapelle JM, Tennstedt D and Marot L. *Atlas of Dermatology*. Brussels, UCB Pharma; 1994.

Sodera V. *Skin Surgery in General Practice. A Diagnostic Atlas.* Bognor Regis, Vija Sodera Publications; 1997.

Very useful for a self-assessment of your diagnostic ability!

White G. *Levene's Colour Atlas of Dermatology* (2e). London, Mosby-Wolfe; 1997.

7

Common cutaneous lesions: pre-malignant and malignant

PRE-MALIGNANT LESIONS

Introduction

Pre-malignant lesions are:

- actinic keratoses (solar keratoses)
- keratoacanthoma
- Bowen's disease.

The choice of treatment is a decision made by the surgeon with the patient after discussing the pros and cons of various methods of treatment. The ultimate method is largely dependent on the equipment and instruments available, the repertoire of skills and experience of the surgeon, and the nature, size and site of the lesion.

Actinic keratoses (solar keratoses)

Actinic keratoses are epidermal neoplasms consisting of altered keratinocytes.[1] Seen in fair-skinned populations, and a higher prevalence in those living near the equator.

Commonly seen in the dorsum of the hands of elderly people, from chronic sun exposure. The rough lesions may be papular or scaly. The size varies from 2 mm to large plaques, although the majority are between 2 and 6 mm in diameter.[2] The lesions could be flesh coloured, pigmented, erythematous or tan. Usually they are reddish-white scaly lesions. Tiny lesions may resolve spontaneously. Actinic keratoses are pre-malignant cutaneous neoplasms showing chromosomal abnormalities that occur primarily on sun-exposed skin surfaces.[2] They **must** be treated to prevent conversion to squamous cell carcinoma (SCC), although only about 0.1% do transform into SCC. If an actinic keratosis converts to a squamous cell carcinoma, it may bleed, ulcerate, become infected, destroy anatomical structures or spread. Sun-protection advice is important as it may prevent the development of further lesions.

Characteristics

- Age: usually after 40. Depends on duration of sun exposure.
- Sex: both males and females.
- Site: sun-exposed areas. Especially dorsum of hands.
- Size: usually 2–6 mm in diameter, though they could be of any size.
- Symmetry: mostly asymmetrical.
- Surface: rough, scaly. Characteristically the surface scale is better felt than seen.
- Border: usually ill-defined.
- Colour: uniformly pink/red in colour. Occasionally pigmented.

Differential diagnosis

Early squamous cell carcinoma in large, solitary lesions; basal cell carcinoma, viral wart and flat seborrhoeic keratosis.

Management

Sun-protection advice is mandatory. Depends on age, number of lesions and whether there has been a recent change in shape, size, colour or symptoms, such as itching and bleeding.

As these lesions are premalignant they **should be treated** to prevent malignant transformation. They could be treated by cryosurgery or excision biopsy.

Cryosurgery

Cannot do histology, but acceptable treatment if diagnosis is clinically certain, by partial incisional biopsy and for multiple lesions.

Excision biopsy

For small, solitary lesion. A clearance of at least a 2 mm margin is recommended. If there are no alarming symptoms or signs, in a very elderly patient, one could **monitor** periodically without any intervention, after baseline observations including measurement and documentation. Ideally a digital or normal photographic record will be most useful. The patient should be counselled regarding symptoms and signs to look for. Continued surveillance is important. This form of *expectant management* should be an exception rather than the rule. Excision of a solitary lesion may be appropriate if diagnosis is uncertain, or if the lesion is papular, suggesting the transformation to squamous cell carcinoma. The usual rule: 'If in doubt – refer' holds true in this situation. Shave excision biopsy followed by a radiosurgical contouring is useful, if available. Alternatively, electrofulgaration is possible.

Topical antimitotic agent

A topical antimitotic agent such as 5-fluorouracil can be used by *dermatologists*. This requires close supervision to prevent complications. Used in patients with multiple lesions. *Refer* the patient to a dermatologist. Dermatologists also use other techniques such as dermabrasion, chemical peels and laser resurfacing.

Keratoacanthoma (molluscum sebaceum)

This is a *rapidly growing* tumour from the pilosebaceous follicles. The history is that the lesion has been growing larger in the previous few weeks.

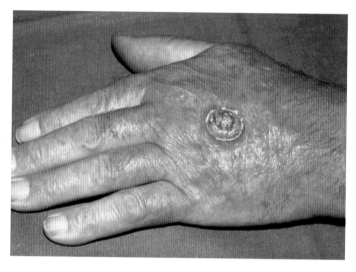

Figure 7.1 Keratoacanthoma on hand (courtesy of Dr C Grattan).

These lesions usually resolve spontaneously over about 3–6 months, if untreated. They are benign by virtue of their typical natural history. However, they are often difficult to differentiate clinically and histologically from squamous cell carcinoma.

Characteristics

- Age: usually more common in middle age than in the elderly.
- Sex: both males and females. Uncommon in dark-skinned races and Japanese.
- Site: anywhere. Usually sun-exposed areas. Commonly in head (face) and upper limbs. Usually a solitary lesion.
- Size: less than 1 cm in maximal diameter, when patient consults.
- Symmetry: symmetrical.
- Surface: papular lesion, with central crater of keratin plug, which is characteristic.
- Border: well-defined, rounded papule. The epidermis over the nodule looks shiny and transparent, with telangiectasiae just visible under the skin. The centre has a horny plug of keratin.
- Colour: uniformly rounded, flesh coloured.

Differential diagnosis

May resemble solitary cutaneous horn, molluscum contagiosum, wart or hypertrophic solar keratosis.

Management

Explain the natural history to the patient, but examine the base of the lesion. If irregular in any way, or if the crater margin is everted, one should exclude an underlying squamous cell carcinoma. *Excision biopsy* is the most appropriate method, to confirm diagnosis. If the lesion is large, a paracentral elliptical excision including the margins and normal skin should be excised for biopsy. Alternatively, a thin radial wedge biopsy, including the centre of the lesion and normal skin beyond the margin, is acceptable. **All** excision biopsy *must include subcutaneous fat*, to ensure that the entire thickness of the lesion is biopsied. Invasion of the deeper dermis is seen in a squamous cell carcinoma, but not in keratoacanthoma. Hence the importance of the depth of the biopsy to include the subcutaneous fat in all biopsies of cutaneous lesions. Lesions on the face could be referred to a plastic surgeon or dermatologist. If the patient refuses intervention, monitor progress periodically, until the entire lesion resolves. This usually takes about 3–6 months. If there is a post-involutional residual scar-like lesion, squamous cell carcinoma must be excluded by excision biopsy including 2 mm wide clearance and subcutaneous fat.

Bowen's disease (intra-epidermal carcinoma *in situ*)

Characteristics

- Age: usually after 40. More common in the elderly.
- Sex: both males and females.
- Site: anywhere, usually sun-exposed areas. Commonly on legs.
- Size: usually more than 1 cm in maximal diameter, when patient consults.
- Symmetry: asymmetrical.
- Surface: maculo-papular, rough scaly plaques.

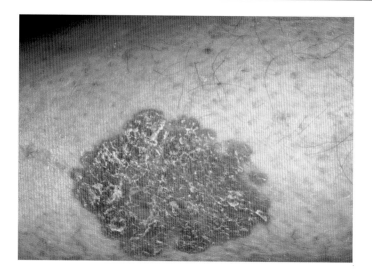

Figure 7.2 Bowen's disease (courtesy of Dr C Grattan).

- Border: usually well-defined, reniform borders.
- Colour: uniformly pigmented, erythematous, tanned or fleshy.

Differential diagnosis

May resemble a solitary eczema or psoriatic patch.

If untreated, may progress to squamous cell carcinoma, and spreads laterally and vertically into dermis and may metastasise. It could take many years to transform into SCC.

MALIGNANT LESIONS

Introduction

For practical purposes, skin cancers could be divided into non-melanoma skin cancers and malignant melanoma.

- Non-melanoma skin cancers:
  - basal cell carcinoma (BCC)
  - squamous cell carcinoma (SCC).
- Malignant melanoma (MM).

As a general rule **all** clinically malignant lesions should be *referred* urgently. Epidemiological studies reveal an increasing incidence of skin cancer, perhaps related to global warming. Primary care plays a pivotal role in the prevention of skin cancer. The primary healthcare team clinicians (PHCT), which includes the family practitioner (general practitioner) and practice nurse (nurse practitioner), the community health carers (including health visitors, community physicians, school nurses, to name but a few) and all health educators have to make a concerted effort, if the *Health of the Nation* targets are to be achieved, especially for skin cancers. The United Kingdom Department of Health objective for skin cancers is: 'To halt the year on year increase in the incidence of skin cancer by the year 2005'.

At least 40 000 new cases of skin cancers are diagnosed each year in the United Kingdom, and the numbers are rising. According to the British Association of Dermatology, 80% of all skin cancers are avoidable. If we wish to halt the increase in incidence and reverse the trend, and thereby reduce morbidity and mortality from skin cancers, our strategies should include three important areas:

☺ Prevention
☺ Early detection
☺ Appropriate management and follow-up.

In all three areas, primary care could have the greatest impact on the objectives. Community-based and practice-based efforts are essential.

How can we maximise prevention?

☺ Discouraging and preventing sunburn.
☺ Encouraging screening.

For effective prevention, we have to *know* who is most at risk for melanoma cancers and non-melanoma cancers.

What are the risk factors for melanoma cancers?

☹ Skin that burns easily, rather than tans (skin types 1 and 2). Previous history of recurrent sunburn.
☹ Family history of dysplastic naevus syndrome.
☹ Family history of malignant melanoma.
☹ Past history of malignant melanoma.
☹ Blonde hair.
☹ Blue eyes.

☹ Multiple freckles.
☹ Multiple dysplastic naevi (>100 benign naevi in young adults; >50 in older adults; or >3 atypical naevi).
☹ Large congenital naevi.

Although all the above risk factors must be considered in an individual, the *majority of malignant melanomas arise de novo and **not** from a pre-existing mole*. In Ackerman's large series of more than 75 000 malignant melanomas in Caucasians, about 80% arose *de novo*.[3] The same author critically appraised the nomenclature of pigmented naevi in the literature, highlighting the lack of definite criteria in describing dysplasia, dysplastic cells, dysplastic naevi, the dysplastic naevus syndrome and atypical mole syndrome. He proposed that they all be called 'common naevi' in the interest of simplicity, accuracy and care of patients. However, the confusion continues a decade later. Furthermore, current trends seem to suggest that the proportion of melanomas arising from a pre-existing mole is nearer 50%.

What are the risk factors for non-melanoma skin cancers?

Basal cell carcinoma

☹ Usually >40 years.
☹ Poor tanners (skin phototypes 1 and 2).
☹ Red hair.
☹ Freckles.
☹ Prolonged ultraviolet exposure.

Squamous cell carcinoma

☹ Usually >40 years.
☹ Many years of ultraviolet exposure.
☹ Pre-malignant lesions such as solar keratosis or Bowen's disease.

The National Cancer Research Campaign suggests the following prevention advice for skin cancers:

• avoid sunburn
• keep babies out of the sun altogether
• protect children from sunburn; sunburn in under-15-year-olds increases the risk of skin cancer later in life
• limit exposure to the sun

- avoid direct sun between 11 a.m. and 3 p.m.
- wear a broad-brimmed hat and cool, loose, but tight-woven clothing in the sun
- use a *sunscreen* with a protection factor (SPF) of >15 *with additional UVA protection*
- don't spend extra time in the sun, even if you use a sunscreen; there is no such thing as a safe tan
- avoid the use of sunbeds.

All health carers, including general practitioners, should disseminate the above information to all their patients.

Early detection

The primary care team has a vital role to play in the professional and public education to ensure prevention and early detection of malignant melanomas.

Professor Rona Mackie

The ways in which this can be achieved are listed below.

- Increasing the awareness of the population about 'mole watch'. Periodic media campaigns are useful. TV, radio, newspapers, large billboard advertising, leaflets, advertising on beaches, waiting-room noticeboards and patient newsletters are some options.
- Increasing the awareness of general practitioners and practice nurses, to examine patients opportunistically.
- Increasing the competence of community clinicians, including GPs and nurses, in diagnosing skin lesions. Clinicians should be able to differentiate clinically between the benign, borderline and malignant lesions, and take appropriate action.
- All GPs should be able to apply the 'seven-point code' for the early detection of malignant melanomas.
- Patients and all other health carers should at least be aware of the three major signs of the 'seven-point code'. This checklist is a useful aid to early diagnosis.

> ## The 'seven-point code'[4] has three major signs and four minor signs
>
> Major signs (the three 'S's of malignant melanoma)
>
> 1   *Increasing* size of an existing mole or *recent appearance* of a new mole.
>
> 2   The mole has an *irregular shape* (asymmetry).
>
> 3   The mole has mixed *shades* of brown and black in colour.
>
> Minor signs
>
> 1   A mole bigger than the blunt end of a pencil (>6 *mm diameter*).
>
> 2   *Inflammation*, with a reddish border.
>
> 3   *Crusting, oozing* or *bleeding*.
>
> 4   Feels different: recent *itching* or *discomfort* or pain.

Action plan for seven-point code

- One or more major signs – consider *urgent referral*.
- Additional presence of one or more minor signs significantly increases the possibility of malignant melanoma.
- Three or more minor signs without major signs – consider referral.
- In your referral letter, include clinical findings, and presence or absence of regional or other lymph nodes, and palpability of liver and spleen.

A, B, C, D, E of malignant melanoma

Another useful concept is the 'A,B,C,D,E'[5] of malignant melanoma:

- ☹ *asymmetry* of the pigmented lesion (corresponds to the *shape* irregularity of the seven-point code)
- ☹ *border* irregularity
- ☹ *colour* irregularity or variegation (corresponds to the *shades* factor of the seven-point code)
- ☹ *diameter* of over 6 mm (corresponds to the *size* factor of the seven-point code)
- ☹ *elevation* above the surface (maculo-papular lesion).

(Although all the above features may also be seen in dysplastic naevi, recent *change* in size, shape and shades of colour is very highly suggestive of malignant melanoma.)

Management issues on all cutaneous lesions

- *Benign lesions*: reassure or remove, depending on symptoms.
- *Probably benign*: remove and send for histology. Follow-up is mandatory. Have a system for follow-up of all lesions sent for histology.
- *Probably malignant*: refer urgently. If you deal with the lesion, ensure at least a 2 mm lateral clearance *and* adequate depth clearance. **Always** send it for histology. Follow-up of patient and histology report is mandatory.
- *Malignant lesions*: immediate, urgent referral. It is quicker to refer immediately by telephone and faxing the referral letter to the consultant, if you are definite of the clinical diagnosis, especially malignant melanoma. If you do an excisional biopsy, ensure at least 2 mm clearance from the margin, with a depth up to the fascia below. It is mandatory to ensure that you have excised the entire width and depth of the lesion by including the subcutaneous fat up to the underlying fascia. *Urgent histology and follow-up is mandatory.*

To whom you refer will depend on local arrangements and the site and nature of the lesion. You may refer to a general surgeon, plastic surgeon or dermatologist. Communication and follow-up is very important. Most histopathology forms have the doctor's contact telephone number, below the signature. It is important to fill this in. It enables the pathologist to contact you immediately if a lesion is malignant and you will have to refer the patient for definitive treatment.

Reflections

- What system of follow-up do you have for checking the histology of lesions sent to the pathology department?

- What is your management protocol for dealing with a histology report which states that a lesion you have sent is a malignant melanoma with a Breslow thickness of 0.74 mm?

Non-melanoma skin cancers

BASAL CELL CARCINOMA (RODENT ULCER)

Who is vulnerable?

☹ The poor tanners.
☹ Those with red hair and freckles.

Characteristics

- Age: usually over 40. Depends on duration of sun exposure. Common in the elderly.
- Sex: both males and females.
- Site: sun-exposed areas, especially the face, near the canthus of the eye, nose.
- Size: usually under 1.5 cm in the maximum diameter.
- Symmetry: mostly symmetrical.
- Surface: smooth, round nodular lesion in the early phase. Surface telangiectasia is common. Cystic BCC has a pearly hue. Stretching the skin enhances this characteristic of the lesion. Ulceration occurs later. When ulcerated, may resemble squamous cell carcinoma.
- Border: usually well-defined, slow growing. Locally malignant. Almost never metastasise.
- Colour: usually pearly hue or skin-coloured. May be pigmented.

Differential diagnosis

Solitary rodent ulcers may resemble SCC. Pigmented lesions may resemble nodular malignant melanoma.

Management

Sun-protection advice is important. Ideally *referred*. Doubtful small lesions are better excised for histological diagnosis, with at least a 2 mm marginal clearance, including the full thickness of the dermis, by including the subcutaneous fat. Long-term follow-up and surveillance for local recurrence and development of new lesions are essential.

SQUAMOUS CELL CARCINOMA

Who is vulnerable?

- ☹ People with sun-damaged skin, from prolonged ultraviolet radiation.
- ☹ Actinic keratoses and keratoacanthoma.
- ☹ Long-term contact with X-rays and infrared rays.
- ☹ Long-term contact with carcinogens such as tar, pitch, mineral oils and inorganic arsenic.
- ☹ Patients with chronic ulcers and scars.

Characteristics

- Age: usually over 40. Depends on duration of sun exposure. Common in the elderly.
- Sex: both males and females.
- Site: sun-exposed areas.
- Size: usually over 1 cm in diameter at the time of diagnosis, although they could be of any size.
- Symmetry: usually asymmetrical.
- Surface: irregular surface. Often ulcer-like lesion.
- Border: asymmetrical, margins are *elevated* and *everted*, typically.
- Colour: depends on the presence or absence of ulceration and bleeding.

Differential diagnosis

Basal cell carcinoma.

Management

Refer for definitive treatment.

Malignant melanoma

Malignant melanoma writes its message in the skin with its own ink and it is there for all of us to see. Some see but do not comprehend.

Neville Davis (1978)

This arises from the epidermal melanocytes. Malignant melanoma incidence is *increasing* all over the world, especially in the white-skinned races. Its prevention, early diagnosis and appropriate management depend on primary care. The primary-care physician needs to be able to give preventive advice for skin cancers, and to diagnose it early, if the patient presents with a pigmented mole which has appeared recently, or changed in size, shape or colour. You should be able to diagnose it opportunistically, when you see any moles while examining a patient for a different complaint. You should be able to differentiate clinically between benign banal melanocytic naevi, atypical and dysplastic naevi, and malignant melanoma. However, in reality this is not always possible. If there are doubts, or if borderline lesions are encountered, it is better to either refer to a dermatological surgeon or to completely excise the lesion with a 2 mm margin and depth to include subcutaneous fat, and send for urgent histology; and follow up the report.

> *There was a big blonde with blue eyes,*
> *Who loved to fly the skies,*
> *She had a small mole that was brown*
> *That moved up and down when she frowned*
> *She laid in the sun,*
> *All just for fun,*
> *And the mole that was brown,*
> *Grew and covered her crown,*
> *It turned into black,*
> *Because she was slack,*
> *In putting on her lotion,*
> *Of which she had no notion*
> *And now she lies with no motion!*

Four types of malignant melanoma are described:

1 lentigo maligna melanoma (mainly on the face of the elderly) (*see* Figure 7.3)
2 superficial spreading malignant melanoma (most common, about 70%) (*see* Figure 7.4)
3 nodular malignant melanoma (vertically growing, aggressive, thick tumour) (*see* Figure 7.5)

4   acral and acral-lentiginous melanoma (palms, soles and around nails) (*see* Figure 7.6).

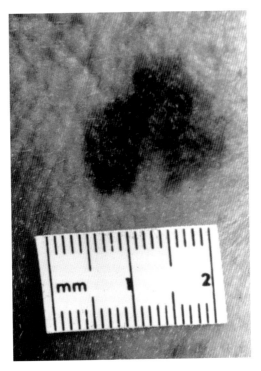

Figure 7.3 Lentigo maligna melanoma (courtesy of Professor R Mackie).

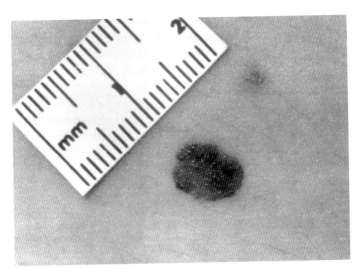

Figure 7.4 Superficial spreading melanoma (courtesy of Dr C Grattan).

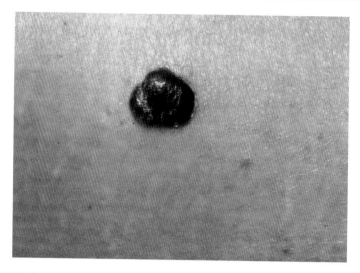

Figure 7.5 Nodular melanoma (courtesy of Professor R Mackie).

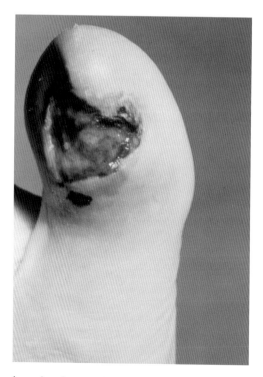

Figure 7.6 Subungual acral melanoma (courtesy of Professor R Mackie).

Characteristics

- Age: usually young and middle age (15–40). Very rare before puberty. Lentigo maligna melanoma occurs at an older age.
- Sex: both males and females; in UK, more common in females.
- Site: sun-exposed areas. In females majority occur on the lower limbs, especially the legs. In males the majority occur on the trunk, especially the back.[6] Females have a better prognosis.
- Size: most malignant melanomas are more than 6 mm in diameter at the time of diagnosis, but unsuspected and borderline lesions excised in primary care are often less than 6 mm.
- Symmetry: usually asymmetrical (the 'A' of the ABCDE of MM).
- Surface: macular, maculo-papular or nodular.
- Border: ill-defined, especially lentigo maligna and superficial spreading melanoma. Margins are abrupt in nodular melanomas, due to the absence of a radial growth phase.
- Colour: usually variegated. Different shades of black, brown and tan colour.

Differential diagnosis

Pigmented basal cell carcinoma, atypical melanoma, dysplastic naevi, some freckles which are darker after sun exposure, seborrhoeic warts and pigmented angiomas. The seven-point checklist and ABCDE rules help to distinguish in the majority, but not all. Amelanotic melanoma is pinkish in colour and resembles pyogenic granuloma. Malignant melanoma may mimic almost any cutaneous lesion. The history and histology help to confirm the diagnosis. In a recent survey in the North-East Thames region of England, it was noted that the general practitioners' diagnostic accuracy of melanomas was low. But only 7% of the melanomas were removed in general practice, and those removed by general practitioners were more likely to be amelanotic.[7] The golden rule is to *excise or refer, if in doubt*. It is known that the diagnostic accuracy of even dermatologists in diagnosing malignant melanoma can be only 50%.[8] A more recent study on the clinical diagnostic accuracy of pigmented skin lesions by consultants and senior and junior registrars, from a pigmented lesion clinic in Glasgow,[9] showed that the two consultants involved in the study (with more than 10 years' experience) had a diagnostic accuracy of 80% for melanoma, compared with 62% for the senior registrar level and 56% for registrar level. Although it was a secondary-care study on a selective group of patients referred to a pigmented lesion clinic, it has implications for primary care. General practitioners should enhance their skills in the *early diagnosis* and appropriate management of pigmented lesions, or refer if they are not able to deal with this. Primary prevention by health education is very important, if we hope to achieve the halt to the increasing incidence of melanomas. Schools, media and health education bodies have an important role. Patients *need to be encouraged to seek help earlier*, for an early diagnosis and management.

Management

Prevention

- Sun protection advice.
- Surveillance of those who have freckles, multiple banal or dysplastic naevi, by whole-body examination or photography periodically.
- Increasing patient awareness about 'mole watch'.
- Surveillance of those patients with a past history of malignant melanoma, which has been treated.

Treatment

Refer urgently all definite malignant melanomas, and stage II or III malignant melanomas.

Small stage I primary cutaneous melanomas – complete excision with at least 2 mm lateral clearance, including the entire thickness of the lesion by ensuring a depth clearance up to the deep fascia, and urgent histology is acceptable. But the *follow-up* and referral for secondary procedures, as soon as possible or within 4 weeks of the primary procedure, is **mandatory**. The delay between the primary limited excision and the secondary, definitive wider excision should **not** exceed a maximum of 4 weeks.

Reflections

- What are the distinguishing features of the different types of melanoma?
- How many skin cancers were diagnosed in the past 3 years in your practice?
- How did the pre-operative clinical diagnoses correlate with the histology?
- What is your practice protocol for the follow-up of lesions sent for histology?

Key issues for primary care of malignant melanoma

- Risk factors and primary prevention: involving the primary healthcare team and public.
- Differential diagnoses and early diagnosis.
- Management of suspicious lesions:
  - importance of width and depth of clearance in narrow margin excision biopsy
  - a system for follow-up of histology and patient
  - self-awareness of competence, and knowing when to refer.
- Management of incompletely excised lesions.
- Prognostic indicators:
  - 'person' factors: ethnicity, age, sex
  - 'lesion' factors: site, type, Breslow thickness, ulceration, mitotic count, vascular invasion, lymphatic invasion, microsatellites, prognostic index.
- Secondary prevention: the follow-up and surveillance of patients who have been treated for malignant melanoma.

Frequently asked questions on malignant melanoma

If a man begins with certainties he shall end in doubts, but if he will be content to begin with doubts he shall end in certainties.

Francis Bacon (1605)

Q. What is the profile of malignant melanomas excised in general practice?

A. A Dutch study[10] demonstrated that in skin biopsies performed by general practitioners, melanomas were mainly detected by chance, and had a very good prognosis as the majority (74%) were small (up to 6 mm) and thin (up to 1.0 mm), although the cohort was small (27 malignant melanomas). Most cutaneous lesions excised in primary care by general practitioners are smaller than 10 mm.

   In a retrospective case-control study conducted in south-east Scotland,[11] 42 malignant melanomas excised by general practitioners over 10 years were analysed. The mean diameter of the lesions excised by general practitioners was significantly less (6.1 mm) than those excised in hospital (9.7 mm). But the Breslow thickness was greater than in the Dutch study, with about 18% having a Breslow thickness of greater than 3 mm. This was similar to the lesions excised in hospital. This study also noted the fact there was no significant difference in the mean time to re-excision for general practitioner and hospital excisions.

Q. Is there any evidence that incomplete lateral excision of a malignant melanoma affects outcome?

A. Currently there is no evidence for this. What matters is the time interval between biopsy in primary care, and definitive treatment in hospital. A comparison of a delay of 21 days between narrow primary excision and delayed definitive wide excision did not show any difference in recurrence rate, or survival at 5 years.[12] Another study also showed that a re-excision within 30 days did not reduce survival time.[13] However, it is essential practice to ensure that *immediate communication* is established with a specialist, on receipt of the histology report, and that the patient is seen by a specialist for definitive treatment *as soon as possible*. Failure to act urgently amounts to negligence. In most hospitals the pathologists contact the general practitioner by telephone, in addition to sending the report. This minimises delay in referral and definitive action.

Q. In primary cutaneous malignant melanoma, will incisional biopsy affect outcome in terms of local recurrence, metastasis or mortality?

A. Lees and Briggs[14] in a review of 1086 patients with stage I cutaneous malignant melanoma concluded that the method of initial biopsy (incisional biopsy, narrow margin excision biopsy and primary wide excision) did *not* affect the prognosis at 5 years' follow-up, in any way. Though incisional biopsy may not affect outcome, the histologist cannot assess the thickest part of the lesion as it may not have been removed. The biopsy scarring may also distort the remaining lesion and make prediction of prognosis difficult. It is therefore important to perform at least an *in toto* excision with at least a 2 mm lateral clearance, and vertical clearance to include a cuff of subcutaneous fat, to ensure that the excision is microscopically complete. Bear in mind that the Breslow thickness is the single most important predictor of prognosis. *Never do a shave biopsy if you suspect a lesion to be a malignant melanoma.*

Q. What should I look for in the histopathology report?

A. The best known pathological feature that affects prognosis is the Breslow thickness. Alexander Breslow[15] described this in 1970. The pathologist's report will usually not only confirm the diagnosis, but also include a statement as to whether the excision was microscopically complete or not. It will also include the *Breslow thickness*, which has implications for prognosis. Absence of *vascular invasion* and the *mitotic count* have an effect on prognosis. *Ulceration*,[16] even if microscopic, is an independent predictor of poor prognosis. Other factors influencing prognosis include *gender* (females have a better prognosis) and *site* of the lesion (back, arms and neck [BAN sites]).

Q. What is Breslow thickness measurement?

A. This is a measurement made by the histopathologist to determine the distance in millimetres between the granular cell layer of the epidermis and the deepest identifiable melanoma cell, using an ocular micrometer. Breslow thickness has been validated as the most useful prognostic indicator for malignant melanoma (Figure 7.7).

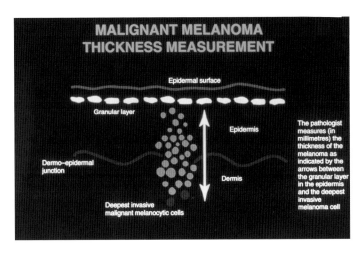

Figure 7.7 Breslow thickness measurement of malignant melanoma.

Q. Why is Breslow thickness measured?

A. Breslow thickness is the best predictor of prognosis. Retrospective and prospective studies have revealed that as the Breslow thickness increases, survival decreases. However, this is not always true. Long-term survival is possible after excising very thick melanomas.[17]

In a prospective study of 1661 patients in Scotland[18] the 5-year survival rates were as follows:

Breslow thickness (mm)	Males (%)	Females (%)
0.1–1.49	84.9	95.4
1.5–3.49	61.8	77.1
>3.5	38	52.9

Breslow, in his own series of 98 patients, noted that *none* had recurrence or metastasis at 5 years, when the thickness of the lesion was less than 0.76 mm.

Q. What is Clark's level of invasion?
A. Clark's level of tumour invasion describes the depth of invasion relative to the skin anatomy:

- level I, malignant melanocytes, confined entirely to the epidermis, i.e. melanoma *in situ*
- level II, minimal invasion of papillary dermis
- level III, invasion and expansion in papillary dermis
- level IV, invasion of reticular dermis
- level V, subdermal invasion.

Q. What is the clinical staging of melanoma?
A.
- Stage I, local tumour only.
- Stage II, regional lymph node involvement.
- Stage III, disseminated disease (metastases +).

Clinical staging and pathological measurements of depth of invasion help the surgeon in planning definitive treatment, and also to assess prognosis.

The resection margins for stage I cutaneous melanoma depend on the tumour thickness. There is controversy on the *width* and *depth* of excision. The resection margins will vary from 2 mm for a melanoma *in situ*, to 3 cm for a tumour that is over 2 mm Breslow thickness. Most surgeons will excise down to the level of the deep fascia. The relevance for the GP is **not** to breach the deep fascia, when excising a pigmented lesion in primary care. Breaching the deep fascia may potentially facilitate the spread of a stage I melanoma. However, there seems to be no research evidence to support this.

The use of magnification in cutaneous lesions

Using magnification to assess skin lesions does help to enhance diagnostic accuracy. The dermatoscope is a hand-held instrument, which looks like an otoscope and provides a skin surface magnification of about ×10.[19] With halogen illumination at an angle of 20°, and oil or disinfecting solution applied to the lesion, the horny layer becomes more translucent.

Reflections

- The incidence of malignant melanoma is increasing.

- The aim of the *Health of the Nation* target is to put a halt to this by the year 2005.

- The primary-care team has a vital role to play in public and professional education, early diagnosis and appropriate management.

- Risk factors include white skin types 1 and 2, which burn and don't tan or tan with difficulty, blonde hair, blue eyes and age between 15 and 40 years.

- In the evolution of a malignant melanoma, the majority (except nodular melanoma) show radial growth before vertical growth.

- The seven-point code and the 'ABCDE' rules help in clinical diagnosis.

- Primary cutaneous malignant melanoma is best referred, or completely excised for biopsy with a margin of at least 2 mm, adequate depth to include a cuff of subcutaneous fat and the histology followed up with subsequent appropriate, urgent action.

- Breslow thickness is the single most important factor in determining prognosis.

- Be a mole watcher! A high index of suspicion in at-risk patients is important.

References

1   Hood AF, Kwan TH, Mihm MC Jr *et al.* Neoplastic patterns of the epidermis. In: ER Farmer and AF Hood (eds) *Primer of Dermatopathology* (2e), pp. 112–15. Boston, Little Brown; 1993.

2   Callen JP, Bickers DR and Moy RL. Actinic keratoses. *J Am Acad Dermatol.* 1997; **36**: 650–3.

3   Ackerman AB. What naevus is dysplastic, a syndrome and the commonest precursor of malignant melanoma? A riddle and an answer. *Histopathol.* 1988; **13**: 241–56.

4   Mackie RM. *Malignant Melanoma. A Guide to Early Diagnosis.* Glasgow, University of Glasgow; 1989.

5   Friedman RJ, Rigel DS and Kopf AW. Early detection of malignant melanoma: the role of physician examination and self-examination of the skin. *Cancer J Clin.* 1985; **35**(3): 130–51.

6   Shaw HM, Milton GW, Farago G and McCarthy WH. Endocrine influences on survival from malignant melanoma. *Cancer.* 1978; **42**: 669–77.

7   Khorshid SM, Pinney E and Newton Bishop JA. Melanoma excision by general practitioners in North-East Thames region, England. *Br J Dermatol.* 1998; **138**: 412–17.

8   Kopf AW, Mintzis M and Bart RS. Diagnostic accuracy in malignant melanoma. *Arch Dermatol.* 1975; **111**: 1291–2.

9   Morton CA and Mackie RM. Clinical accuracy of the diagnosis of cutaneous malignant melanoma. *Br J Dermatol.* 1998; **138**: 283–7.

10   Bosch MM and Boon ME. Profile of the malignant melanoma excised in general practice. *Br J Dermatol.* 1994; **130**(1): 57–61.

11   Herd RM, Hunter JAA, McLaren KM, Chetty U, Watson ACH and Gollock JM. Excision biopsy of malignant melanoma by general practitioners in south east Scotland 1982–91. *BMJ.* 1992; **305**: 1476–8.

12   Landthaler M, Braun-Falco O, Leitl A, Konz B and Holzer D. Excision biopsy as the first therapeutic procedure versus primary wide excision of malignant melanoma. *Cancer.* 1989; **64**: 1612–16.

13   Lederman JS and Sober AJ. Does biopsy type influence survival in clinical stage 1 cutaneous melanoma? *J Am Acad Dermatol.* 1985; **13**: 983–7.

14   Lees VC and Briggs JC. Effect of initial biopsy procedure on prognosis in Stage 1 invasive cutaneous malignant melanoma: review of 1086 patients. *Br J Surg.* 1991; **78**: 1108–10.

15   Breslow A. Thickness, cross-sectional areas and depth of invasion in the prognosis of cutaneous melanoma. *Ann Surg.* 1970; **172**: 902–8.

16   Balch CM, Wilkerson JA, Murad TM *et al.* The prognostic significance of ulceration of cutaneous melanoma. *Cancer.* 1980; **45**: 3012–17.

17   Blessing K, McLaren KM, McLean A and Davidson P. Thick malignant melanomas (>3 mm Breslow) with good clinical outcome: a histological study and survival analysis. *Histopathol.* 1991; **18**: 143–8.

18   Mackie R, Hunter JA, Aitchison TC *et al.* Cutaneous malignant melanoma. Scotland 1979–89. *Lancet.* 1992; **339**: 971–5.

19   Stolz W, Bilek P, Landthaler M *et al.* Skin surface microscopy. *Lancet.* 1989; **2**: 864–5.

Further reading

Havlik RJ, Vakasin AP and Ariyan S. The impact of stress on the clinical presentation of melanoma. *Plast Reconst Surg.* 1991; **90**: 57–61.

Mackie RM. *Malignant Melanoma. A Guide to Early Diagnosis*. Edinburgh, Pillans & Wilson; 1994.

McEldowney S. Malignant melanoma: familial, genetic, and psychosocial risk factors. *Clin Rev.* 1997; 7(7): 65–8, 73–6, 81–2.

8

Freeze or fry?

Cryotherapy

According to Zacarian,[1] the use of 'cold' in a controlled way for the selective destruction of components of cutaneous lesions has been used since 1877. The main advantage of cryotherapy is the good cosmetic result, as scarring is minimal if used judiciously. It is relatively pain free, and convenient for patient and doctor. Multiple lesions could be treated in one sitting. Most patients could return to work on the same day or next day. Cryotherapy does not require an anaesthetic or sterility. It is inexpensive and carried out effectively in the surgery.

The main disadvantage is the storage and filling of cryogen. It is stored in special storage Dewars with a liquid nitrogen withdrawal device. The static holding time of the Dewars varies with their capacity. Once liquid nitrogen is transferred to canisters, it has to be used in 12–24 hours. You will need to have about 5–15 patients in one sitting for it to be worthwhile. It may not be cost-effective to treat one or two patients at a time. Smaller practices could consider the use of a Histofreezer, as the shelf-life is much longer, avoiding the problem of having to fill the canister with the cryogen, usually from the local hospital. Cryotherapy is not useful for hairy areas, as the hair follicles are destroyed, and will not regrow. Another disadvantage is that tissue cannot be sent for biopsy, as it will be destroyed by the cold. Furthermore, in brown- and black-skinned people, hypopigmentation will be marked as melanocytes are the most sensitive cells to cryotherapy. Although healing is cosmetically good on white skin, the healed site is prone to sunburn, and will need sunscreen creams. Complications, although rare, could occur. These include damage to underlying tissues such as cartilage, tendon or superficial nerves, or haemorrhage and infection.

If you have never used cryotherapy, it would be wise to attend a training course, and to practise on a pig's trotter or tomatoes. Observing and practising under supervision in a cryotherapy clinic is most useful if you intend to use cryotherapy.

See one,
Do one,
Teach one.

An old surgical maxim. Perhaps the 'one' should be replaced by 'some'!

Cryogens

- Liquid nitrogen: commonly used in primary care. Since it boils at –196°C, it is stored in containers that allow evaporation. Liquid nitrogen is used in equipment such as the Cry-AC, Cryojem and Cryojet with the spray or probe technique. Zacarian[2] devised the hand-held units for cryotherapy. The use of liquid nitrogen in cotton-wool buds is obsolete. The depth to which it is effective is very minimal.
- Dimethyl-ether and propane aerosol (Histofreezer).
- Nitrous oxide: used in colposcopy and genito-urinary clinics and ENT clinics. The temperature reached is about –85°C and can be applied only with a probe.

Of the above, liquid nitrogen and dimethyl-ether and propane aerosol are the commonly used cryogens. The accessories used with the liquid nitrogen hand-held canister include: spray tips of varying sizes, probes, spray-limiting neoprene cones and protective items such as adhesive putty.

Principle and mechanism

Sub-zero freezing of cells destroys the lesion by two methods: a direct effect on the cells and the vascular stasis that occurs after thawing. Further damage occurs as a result of the effect of freezing on the microcirculation. Rapid freezing of the target tissue followed by slow thawing ensures optimal destruction. The freeze time will depend on the technique used, size, depth, nature and location of the lesion. Maximal destruction occurs with repeated freeze–thaw cycles. A second freeze–thaw cycle has been shown to kill all the cells of the skin. Usually collagen fibres and cartilage are resistant to destruction. Hence healing occurs without cosmetic disfigurement. Healing is by secondary intention.

The reaction that results from freezing includes erythema, oedema, vesiculation, exudation and sloughing with eschar formation.[3] It takes about 1–2 weeks for the wound to dry.

Indications

Benign lesions

This is the main indication, *unless* one has extensive cryosurgical experience.

☺ Viral warts are the most common lesions treated by cryotherapy. The aim of treatment should be to raise a bulla, caused by separation of the dermo-epidermal junction, which extends further lateral to the lesion. The freezing time will depend on the thickness of the lesion and the technique. May need more than one treatment. Also very useful for peri-ungual lesions.
☺ Seborrhoeic warts.
☺ Skin tags/fibroepitheliomas.
☺ Molluscum contagiosum.
☺ Mucoid cysts.
☺ Dermatofibromas.
☺ Pyogenic granuloma.
☺ Cherry angiomas.
☺ Chondrodermatitis nodularis helicis.

☺ Solar lentigo.
☺ Lentigines.

Pre-malignant and malignant lesions

Best referred unless you have the experience and expertise to deal with them. Bowen's disease is often treated by cryotherapy, especially after histological confirmation of diagnosis. The target for the coldest temperature at the base of a malignancy must be at least −50°C, to freeze the skin completely, if and when you treat basal cell or squamous cell carcinomas. Basal cell carcinoma and squamous cell carcinoma may be treated by cryotherapy in secondary care. Malignant melanoma should **never** be treated by cryosurgery in primary care. *All skin cancers are better managed in secondary care.*

Contraindications

☹ Lesions where histology is important, e.g. malignant lesions such as melanoma. You will not be able to confirm the diagnosis once the lesion is destroyed by cryotherapy. It would be *medically negligent* to treat a malignant melanoma by cryotherapy.
☹ Proven allergy or hypersensitivity to cryogens, as in immunocompromised diseases, known cold urticaria or cold intolerance.
☹ Patients with cryoglobulinaemia.
☹ Unacceptability of depigmentation by dark-skinned patients.
☹ From the perspective of primary care: any lesion that is definitely not benign. All 'doubtful' and malignant lesions are best referred to a dermatologist or appropriate specialist in secondary care.

Techniques of freezing

Cryospray technique

OPEN SPRAY
Commonly used for benign lesions anywhere except the face. The canister must be held steady, at the appropriate distance from the lesion, to ensure that the ice ball extends about 1–2 mm beyond the margins of the lesion. Having selected a spray button of suitable diameter, commence spraying initially from a distance of 1–2 cm from the surface, steadying the

canister with both hands if needed. The spray is applied intermittently in 2–3 second bursts. The duration will depend on the age of the patient, and size and thickness of the lesion. The maximum duration for children is about 15 seconds. The ice ball needs to be at least 1 mm beyond the margin of the lesion. The ice ball (also called frost ball) should be maintained for about 30 seconds. Adhesive putty can be used to localise the lateral spread from the spray.

CLOSED-CONE TECHNIQUE
More commonly used on the face, ears and other areas where localised freezing limiting lateral spread and depth is important. Alternatively adhesive putty could be used to limit lateral spread.

CRYOPROBE TECHNIQUE
The appropriate sized tip needs to be selected, depending on the size of the lesion. The tip must be clean and dry. The lesion should be covered with K-Y jelly or any lubricant jelly. The freeze time is longer than for the spray technique, usually 30–60 seconds. Remember that the probe will not detach from the lesion, until it has thawed, which will be another 30–60 seconds. It will be wise to elevate the lesion and skin with the probe attached, a few seconds after starting treatment, to prevent damage to underlying structures such as tendons, nerves, blood vessels and joints.

The adequacy of the freezing can also be determined by observing the 'halo thaw time'[4] which is the time taken for surface thawing of the area beyond the lesion. This is usually about 60 seconds, which signifies the adequacy of the ice ball.

Points to consider

- Are you sure of the clinical diagnosis? If you are not definite, refer.
- What are the chances of the lesion being something different, histologically?
- Is it better treated by any other method?
- What is the depth and width of tissue to be frozen?
- Will you have to de-bulk the lesion before freezing?
- Have you explained the procedure, including possible outcomes, and obtained consent?
- What are the three factors determining success? (Freeze time, thaw time and the lateral spread of the ice ball, which should ideally be

about 1–3 mm beyond the edge of the lesion, depending on the nature; 1–2 mm is sufficient for benign lesions.)

Equipment

Cry-AC

Available in 300 ml and 500 ml liquid nitrogen containers with trigger. Adjustable sprays and probes are available as accessories. It is very convenient. The main disadvantage is the short holding time for the cryogen, requiring the organisation of a 'session' of many patients to be cost-effective.

Cryojet

Available as a 500 ml liquid nitrogen canister with trigger. Like Cry-AC, various spray and probe accessories are available.

Histofreezer

Useful for smaller practices. Contains a gas mixture of dimethyl-ether and propane in a 150 ml aerosol canister. The pack comes with 50 2 mm small applicators or 40 5 mm medium applicators.

The applicator can reach a temperature of −57°C. The sensitivity of different types of skin cells varies to cryotherapy. Keratinocytes are far more sensitive than collagen fibres. Melanocytes are also very sensitive to cold destruction. Hence hypopigmentation is a common problem. On the other hand, there is potentially very little scarring, as collagen is quite resistant to cryogens.

The advantage of the Histofreezer is the long shelf-life, about 3 years. But it is inflammable, and should not be used with diathermy. It should be used **only** for *benign lesions*. It is useful for general practitioners who will use cryotherapy for treating benign lesions, and tend to use it sporadically on isolated patients over a period of time. This will be relevant to smaller practices. When treating verrucae and warts, it is important to use a keratolytic wart paint and pumice stone or emery file, to reduce the excrescence of the wart above the skin level, before using the Histofreezer. This helps the penetration and the number of treatments required. Pare down thicker warts before using the Histofreezer. One or two freeze–thaw cycles are used at each session. The freezing time is usually about 40 seconds. The ice ball, seen as whiteness around the lesion, should extend for about 1–2 mm beyond the margins of the lesions. The depth of penetration is usually only up to about 3 mm.

Further information can be obtained from the website: *http://www. histofreezer.com* or email: *info@histofreezer.com*

Complications of cryotherapy

Cryotherapy results in temporary sequelae such as pain, erythema, oedema and blisters, but the incidence of complications is low. It is important to distinguish between the two. Permanent complications often result from inappropriate selection of lesions, patients or poor technique. Knowledge of the anatomy of the region to be treated allows you to predict the possibilities, and counsel the patient accordingly.

Early complications

Common outcomes in bold.

- **Pain,** usually during and just after treatment; temporary.
- Syncopy.
- Headache.
- **Erythema,** usually disappears within a few days.
- **Oedema,** usually mild. Topical or oral steroids could be used for severe oedema and blistering.
- **Blisters.**
- Sepsis.
- Raynaud's phenomenon.
- Severe reaction – in cryoglobulinaemia.
- Injury to tendon, with weakness and rupture. This is uncommon but can also occur as a late complication.
- Paraesthesia in nerves close to treatment area. Usually temporary and does not last beyond 6 weeks.

Late complications

- **Hypopigmentation.**
- Hyperpigmentation.
- Alopecia.
- Nerve injury; usually superficial nerves.
- Injury to cartilage.
- Scarring and permanent retraction of tissues can occur. This includes the eyebrow areas, alae nasi and angle of the mouth when lesions are treated in these areas.

Reflections

- Ensure that you choose the appropriate lesion and the patient for cryotherapy. Consider the five 'A's (age, associated illnesses, allergies, anxiety, anticoagulants).

- Always explain to the patient about the procedure and possible short-term and long-term outcomes.

- Written consent is good practice.

- Reinforce by written instructions on what to expect, and how to manage pain and blisters. If the nurse does the follow-up, have a protocol regarding the indications for the nurse to refer to you.

- Ensure that the equipment is checked and available, with the canisters filled with liquid nitrogen, on the day of the treatment session.

- It will be useful to follow up the patient to assess outcomes, at least once after completing treatment. This is usually about 3 or 4 weeks after treatment.

Cautery

The current use of cautery is more to complement the use of curettage and shave biopsy, to fry the base, and stop bleeding. The equipment used for cautery in primary care includes the following.

- C28 Warecrest cautery equipment (*see* Chapter 3). This is a common instrument used for cautery in primary care. Cautery units can be used in patients with a pacemaker. Cannot control the extent of thermal damage to tissues.
- Other cautery units with step-down transformer and various tips are available, but caution is required if the patient has a pacemaker.
- Hyfrecator (*see* Chapter 3). It *cannot* be used for cutting. Could be used for electrodessication and electrofulguration. It is also used for coagulation. *Avoid using in patients with pacemakers*. It causes a lesser degree of thermal damage to tissues, as it is more controllable.
- Ellman's radiosurgical equipment (*see* Chapter 3). An excellent instrument to use for electrosectioning. Needs practice and acquired

skills to operate efficiently. It is more versatile than the hyfrecator. It can be used for electrosectioning. It is *not* a cautery instrument, as the electrode does not produce heat to destroy tissues. Radio-surgery causes the least damage to tissues, allowing one to achieve maximum control of lateral heat. *Avoid using in patients with pacemakers.*

Indications

Benign lesions

SKIN TAGS

The easiest and quickest way of treating skin tags, especially thin pedunculated lesions, is by cautery with a C28. It does not require an anaesthetic, and takes seconds to treat. This could be done during a consultation and is therefore very convenient. If the base is more than 1–2 mm, a local anaesthetic will be required. In the anxious patient, a topical anaesthetic such as Emla® or Ametop® gel could be used. It is not easy to cauterise flush with the skin. Radiosurgery has a greater cosmetic benefit, as it is possible to excise the lesion with a cutting or cut/coag wave form at a power setting of about 3, and then to achieve haemostasis and plane the base, flush with the surrounding skin, using the coagulation ball electrode. Alternatively, one could fulgarate the base with a fine electrode by alternating fulgaration and wiping with a wet saline swab.

WARTS AND VERRUCAE

These could be treated by cautery, although they are usually treated by cryotherapy, without anaesthetic and the diagnosis is often obvious.

BENIGN PEDUNCULATED LESIONS

Benign pedunculated lesions such as papillomas can be excised by cautery, using local anaesthetic for the base.

Contraindications

Do not use the usual cautery equipment (C28 or the hyfrecator) to remove any pigmented lesions. You may unexpectedly remove a melanoma. The heat destroys the cells and distorts the interpretation by the histologist.

Radiosurgical cautery does not distort the histology and gives a clean cut. Radiosurgery allows one to take a biopsy specimen before proceeding to remove the rest of the lesion.

The main complication of hot cautery is unacceptable scarring, from charring and fibrosis, if used for excision of large lesions. Currently, removal of skin tags is the most common use for cautery. Other lesions are better dealt with by electrocautery or radiosurgery.

Techniques used for biopsy of lesions

Biopsy techniques used in minor surgery:

1   incision biopsy
2   excision biopsy
3   curettage
4   shave and saucerisation biopsy
5   punch biopsy.

See Chapter 10 for 1 and 2. Incision biopsy is usually performed for large lesions or for a large macular rash where diagnosis is uncertain. Excision biopsy is a therapeutic and diagnostic procedure, where the entire lesion is excised.

Curettage

If you want to converse with me, define your terms.
Voltaire (1694–1778)

Curettage is defined as the scraping, scooping or cleansing of a lesion by means of a curette for the removal of new growths or other abnormal tissues.[5] This is a technique of excising an entire lesion, under local anaesthetic, by using a sharp, cutting spoon or ring instrument. The instruments are available as sterilisable and re-usable metallic instruments (e.g. Boyd's or Volkmann's curettes) or single-use, pre-sterilised ring curettes (e.g. Stiefel's ring curettes).

Re-usable spoon curettes

The commonly used curettes come in different sized spoons, either at one end or both ends. Small, medium and large spoon curettes are available, which can be chosen depending on the lesion. These metallic instruments can be sterilised.

Disposable ring curettes

The Stiefel ring curettes come in 4 mm and 7 mm sizes, and can be used for most lesions. The great advantage is that they are single use, and can be discarded after use. Potential for cross-infection is obviated. They are convenient as they come pre-sterilised and are sharp, unlike the spoon curettes, which may become blunt with repeated use. However, they have a limited shelf-life and are more expensive, and one has to consider cost if the service is being provided free to the patient.

Technique of curettage

- Local anaesthetic is required.
- The lesion must be steadied, by using the non-dominant hand, between index finger and thumb. This stabilises the lesion to be curetted.
- Two techniques are commonly used. Depending on the way the instrument is held and used, they are called the pencil technique and the potato-peeler technique.[5] The pencil technique is good for crumbly lesions that don't require strength. In the potato-peeler technique, the thumb does not hold the curette, and is used in addition to the non-dominant hand to stabilise the lesion, by providing tension at a different angle. A third way is to use the thenar eminence and thumb too, to hold the instrument when even greater strength is required to scoop out large, hard solitary warts or verrucae. I call it the golf-club technique.

Indications

The main indication for curettage is in the treatment of benign lesions, especially those that are papular. Seborrhoeic warts, verrucae and molluscum contagiosum could be treated by curettage. Always consider the suitability of other treatment modalities. Bleeding is minimal when friable-looking seborrhoeic warts in the older patient are curetted.

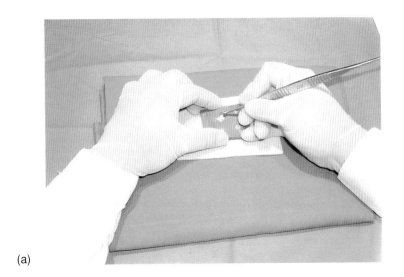

(a)

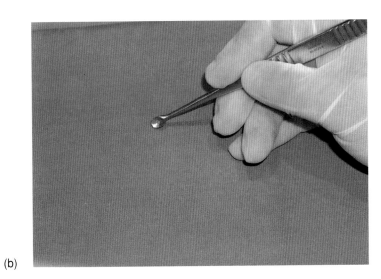

(b)

Figure 8.1 'Pencil' curettage: (a) technique and (b) grip.

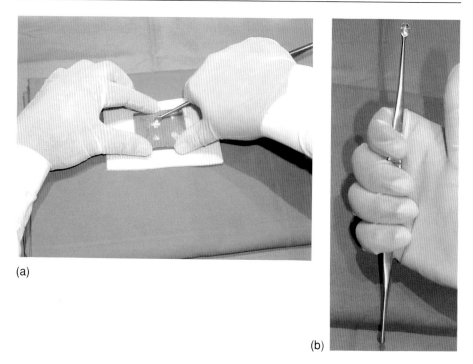

(a)

(b)

Figure 8.2 'Potato peeler' curettage: (a) technique and (b) grip.

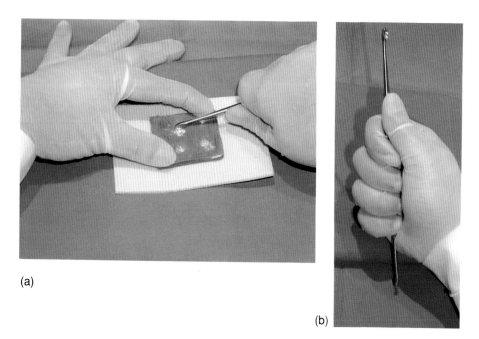

(a)

(b)

Figure 8.3 'Golf club' curettage: (a) technique and (b) grip.

Shave and saucerisation biopsy

Shaving is done by using a sharp knife, parallel to the plane of the skin, via the base of the lesion which is elevated by injecting a local anaesthetic, which produces a wheal. This lifts the lesion slightly above the plane of the skin. The lesion is stabilised between two fingers of the non-dominant hand. Using a size 15 blade on a Bard–Parker handle, the lesion is shaved off the skin by holding the blade parallel to the skin surface, and gradually shaving off the lesion using a gently sawing movement, while lifting the lesion with a Gillies hook, which helps to steady the lesion.

Saucerisation is where the base of the defect is like a crater after the lesion has been removed. This happens more commonly, though not intentionally, when using the Ellman radiosurgical loops to take a biopsy by excising. This can also happen when the blade is not parallel to the skin, but tilted down a little, after entry via the skin. An alternative method is to use one edge of a double-edged Gillette razor blade. This technique is used for the diagnosis and treatment of deeper cutaneous lesions, such as keratoacanthoma.

Punch biopsy

In punch biopsy a cylindrical cutting instrument is used to do an excision or even incision biopsy. The great advantage is that one does not have to plan the placing of the incisions, since on removal of the cylindrical plug of tissue, the remaining defect automatically becomes oval along the relaxed skin tension lines. This makes it easier to apply Steri-strips® or to suture the defect for optimal cosmetic results. The disposable biopsy punch made by Stiefel comes in six different diameters: 2 mm, 3 mm, 4 mm, 5 mm, 6 mm and 8 mm. They are designed to provide a specimen of 2 mm depth. Stiefel ring curettes and biopsy punches come in boxes of ten individually packed curettes and punches.

Technique

- Local anaesthetic is required.
- The lesion needs to be steadied with the non-dominant hand, between thumb and index finger, by applying a stretching tension.
- The punch is applied vertically and turned clockwise and anticlockwise while exerting controlled pressure (be conscious of the anatomy under the lesion!). Once you have gone as far as the base of the lesion

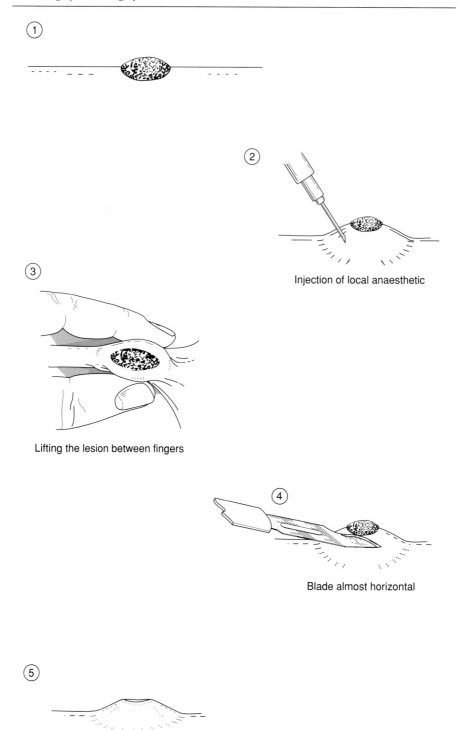

Figure 8.4 Steps in shaving and saucerisation of a benign cutaneous lesion.

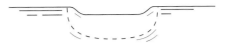

Figure 8.5 Deeper saucerisation.

(don't go drilling too far!), free the lesion by a rocking movement and lift the lesion with a Gillies hook. The excess tissue underneath can be cut off with a sharp scissors. The lesion is sent for histology in a fixative, as usual.

- The defect usually turns oval along the relaxed skin tension lines, and can be closed with Steri-strips® or sutured.

References

1   Zacarian SA. *Cryosurgery for Skin Cancer and Cutaneous Disorders*, pp. 1–30. St Louis, Mosby; 1985.

2   Zacarian SA. Cryotherapy in dermatologic disorders and in the treatment of skin cancer. *J Cryosurg.* 1968; **1**: 70–5.

3   Elton MD. The course of events following cryosurgery. *J Dermatol Surg Oncol.* 1977; **3**: 448–51.

4   Torre D. Depth dose in cryosurgery. *J Dermatol Surg Oncol.* 1983; **9**: 219–25.

5   Adam JE. The technique of curettage surgery. *J Am Acad Dermatol.* 1986; **5**(4): 697–702.

Further reading

Dawber R, Colver G and Jackson A. *Cutaneous Cryosurgery*. Second edition. London, Martin Dunitz; 1997.

Kuflik EG. Cryosurgery updated. *J Am Acad Dermatol.* 1994; **31**(6): 925–44.

Pollack SV. *Electrosurgery of the Skin*. New York, Churchill Livingstone; 1991.

9

Sutures and suturing

Overview

- Introduction.
- Types of sutures.
- Ideal suture material.
- Sutures available on the FP10.
- Techniques:
  - handling the needle holder
  - holding the needle
  - technique of entry and exit
  - simple sutures
  - vertical mattress sutures
  - subcuticular sutures
  - removal of sutures
  - Gillies three-point suturing technique.

Sutures

Sutures (Latin, *sutura* from *suo* = to sew) have been used for thousands of years, to bring together tissues. The technique of suturing is more important in determining the outcome than the actual suture material. This technique can only be learnt by observing the actual procedure or a video teaching aid, followed by practice with animal or simulated materials and, finally, doing it under supervision.

In primary care, the majority of wound closure is achieved by suturing, or using Steri-strips® or both. Skin staples and tissue glue are not usually used. Non-inclusion in the drug tariff and expense precludes the use of skin staples in general practice. The purpose of a suture is to appose the cut edges of a wound until it is sufficiently healed to withstand the tension and separating forces that act on it. The suture will be redundant once this purpose is achieved. The time taken to achieve this will vary in different parts of the human anatomy. For example, wounds of the head and neck heal quicker.

The ideal suture material:

- is easy to handle
- has excellent tensile strength
- stretches when there is oedema and inflammation
- regains its original length when the oedema settles
- is non-reactive, causing hardly any inflammation
- forms a secure knot that will not slip
- does not promote infection
- if buried, should fully dissolve by 4–6 weeks.

There is no material that can achieve all these in the real world. But coated polyglactin (Vicryl®), and polybutester (Novafil®) come close to this ideal. However, they are expensive and not available on prescription.

Some of the causes of early loss of apposition are due to:

- wound inflammation and oedema, leading to sutures cutting through, especially when placed too close to the edges
- wound infection
- breaking of the suture, if too small a thickness is used for high-tension areas
- slipping of the knot, especially with monofilament material, or inadequate tying of the knot
- sutures being absorbed too quickly, when absorbable suture materials are used
- if sutures are removed too quickly before wound healing has been fully established, especially in mobile skin surfaces that are subjected to tension by movement (e.g. the back).

As mentioned in Chapter 10, it is important to ensure the good atraumatic apposition of the various layers, including the skin. Reversed cutting needles prevent the suture material cutting through the edge – if it has been placed too close to the edge. It is wise to place the suture at least 5 mm from the edge, if possible. Tying the knots too tight can also promote cutting through when wound healing occurs with swelling and inflammation.

Classification of suture materials

Suture materials are classified as *absorbable* or *non-absorbable*.

Non-absorbable suture materials

- Silk (derived from thread spun by the silkworm larvae and is braided). Available on the drug tariff (Table 9.1). Excellent handling and knotting qualities, but causes a tissue reaction second to catgut. It has very low tensile strength and, since it is braided, it has a higher potential for promoting infection.
- Polyamide (nylon/Ethilon®). Very commonly used in general practice. It causes minimal tissue reaction and, being a monofilament, does not facilitate infection; it has high tensile strength and is cheap. But extra throws are needed to achieve a secure knot that will not slip. 3/0, 4/0 and 6/0 polyamide as Ethilon® (Table 9.1) are available on prescription.
- Polypropylene (Prolene®). Commonly used in general practice. Both polyamide and Prolene® have good tensile strength, and a low tissue coefficient (able to glide through tissues easily) and cause little tissue reaction. But the knots can slip and therefore extra throws with careful knot placement are essential. Good for subcuticular suturing. Prolene® costs more than nylon, and only one size (4/0) is available on prescription.
- Polybutester (Novafil®). Synthetic, monofilament suture. Does not have significant 'memory' and is therefore easier to manipulate than Prolene® or nylon. Has the unique capacity to elongate or stretch with wound oedema, and regain its original shape after the swelling subsides.

Table 9.1 Suture materials available on the drug tariff

Code	Product description	Size
W507	6/0 Ethilon® (polyamide)	15 mm slimblade
W319	4/0 Ethilon®	19 mm curved reverse-cutting needle
W320	3/0 Ethilon®	26 mm curved reverse-cutting needle
W539	4/0 Prolene®	25 mm slimblade
W501	4/0 Mersilk®	16 mm curved cutting needle
W533	3/0 Mersilk®	25 mm supercutting curved needle
W321	2/0 Mersilk®	26 mm curved reverse-cutting needle
W548	4/0 chromatic catgut	16 mm curved round-bodied needle

- Other non-absorbable sutures *not* usually used in primary care include:
  - linen
  - cotton
  - polyester (Dacron®)
  - stainless steel.

Silk, polyamide and polypropylene are available on the drug tariff, and therefore prescribable.

Absorbable suture materials

- Catgut (plain and chromic – made from animal intestine). It is mammalian collagen derived from the submucosa of sheep intestine or serosa of beef intestine, or the flexor tendons of beef. Chromic catgut is used for suturing episiotomy wounds in primary care, and 4/0 size chromic catgut is available on prescription. Vicryl® is an alternative.
- Polyglycolic acid (Dexon®). Synthetic braided suture. Rather unpredictable absorption.
- Polyglactin (Vicryl®). Synthetic braided suture. Less reactive than Dexon®, excellent knotting and handling. Being coated, eases passage via tissues. Better tensile strength than Dexon®. Undyed Vicryl® should be used, as the dyed type tends to tattoo wounds.
- Polydioxanone (PDS). Monofilament absorbable suture. Longer absorption time and retention of tensile strength.

Remember

Suture materials could be:

- absorbable or non-absorbable

- synthetic or biological/natural

- monofilament or braided.

Figure 9.1 gives a summary of suture materials.

Absorbable suture materials are used for closure of subcutaneous planes, for subcuticular suturing and even skin closure. Sutures nowadays come in pre-sterilised packs. They are either sterilised by γ-irradiation or by using ethylene oxide gas.

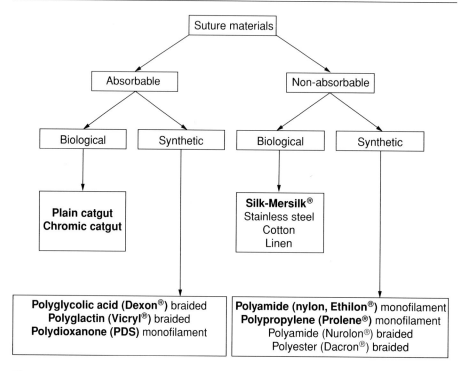

Figure 9.1 Suture materials (those in bold are available on the drug tariff).

The preferred suture sizes for different locations are given in Table 9.2. The actual choice of size is determined by factors such as the thickness of the skin, the tension and the mobility of the area.

All sutures have the following properties, which determine their choice by the surgeon.

- Size. To remove confusion and aid communication both imperial and metric systems are used, as approved by the United States Pharmacopoeia and the European Pharmacopoeia. Both systems will be seen on the front of suture packs. For example, a 3/0 material gauge will also show 2 metric scale gauge on the pack.

Table 9.2 Preferred suture sizes for different locations

Location	Suture size
Face	5/0 or 6/0
Head, scalp	3/0 or 4/0
Neck	4/0 or 5/0
Upper limb	4/0 or 5/0
Trunk and lower limb	3/0 or 4/0

- Tensile strength. In practical terms this is the force required to break a suture.
- Tissue reaction. The synthetic monofilament materials cause the least tissue reaction. The braided, biological materials (silk) or monofilament natural materials cause the most reaction.
- Handling properties and knotting properties. Braided sutures are better than monofilament, synthetic materials.
- Absorption. Absorbable sutures are either destroyed by enzymatic degradation, as in catgut, or hydrolysed, as in polyglactin (Vicryl®) or polydioxanone (PDS).

The absorption rate and duration of tensile strength retention are given in Table 9.3.

Table 9.3 Absorption rate and duration of tensile strength retention of sutures

Suture	Absorption rate (days)	Retention of tensile strength
Plain catgut	5–10	4–5 days
Chromic catgut	90	21–28 days
Polyglycolic acid (Dexon®)	90–120	20% in 14 days 5% in 28 days
Polyglactic acid (Vicryl®)	60–90	60% in 14 days 30% in 21 days
Polydioxanone (PDS)	210	70% in 14 days 50% in 21 days

Needles

The anatomy of a needle

Almost all needles these days are the atraumatic variety. They do not have an eye that needs to be threaded with the suture material. There is hardly any situation where a traumatic needle will be needed in primary-care surgery. All suture needles, whether straight or curved, have a proximal *swaged end* where the suture material is inserted (atraumatic), the *body* of the needle and the *distal inserting end*, which is the cutting or reverse-cutting end. A round-bodied needle, which is useful for suturing deep fat, has little use in most primary-care surgery. The straight needles are useful but not essential for subcuticular suturing.

When holding the needle with a needle holder, ensure that the jaws of the holder are not too near the tip or distal end. This will prevent taking a good 'bite'. On the other hand, if it is held too close to the swaged end (thread end), the needle may bend or break when taking a bite. The optimal place to hold is about two-thirds of the way from the tip of the needle, on the body.

Curved needles can be 3/8 curve, semicircular, or 5/8 curved in shape. Lengths also vary. The standard 'curved' needles have a 3/8 curvature, which is three-eighths of a circle. All the needles available on prescription are 3/8 curvature needles.

Semantics of needles

- Cutting needle: needle with triangular cross-section at the inserting tip, where the apex of the triangle is *inside* the cutting circle. If the 'bite' is taken too close to the edge, the tendency to 'cut through' the skin is greater (compare with the reverse-cutting needle).
- Reverse-cutting needle: this is the same as the cutting needle in shape, but the apex of the triangle is on the outer curvature of the needle. Hence, when taking a bite close to the skin edge the chances of cutting through the edge are less at the time of surgery or subsequently when there is oedema.
- Round-bodied needle: the entire length of the needle is round in cross-section and the distal inserting tip is honed into a conical point.
- Slimblade needle: these are fine-gauge cutting needles.
- P needle: this has a squared cross-section which makes it quite resistant to bending, and easier to push through the skin.

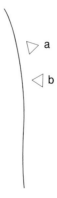

Figure 9.2 Profile of (a) reverse cutting and (b) cutting, with needle placed near the wound edge.

Reflections

Get hold of a suture pack, and look at the information on the front of the pack.

- What information do you find regarding the needle?

- What information do you find regarding the suture material?

- What is an atraumatic needle?

- What is the difference between a cutting and reverse-cutting needle?

- What suture material and needle will you use to remove a sebaceous cyst from the scalp?

- What suture material and needle will you use to remove a lesion from the middle of the back?

- What suture material and needle will you use to remove a lesion from the forearm?

Suturing techniques

The art of suturing should be taught on pieces of cloth, skin or hide.

Sushruta (*c*. 600 BC)

The technique of suturing can only be learnt under supervision. Observing a video helps to facilitate this. An effective method is to observe a demonstration under close-circuit TV, in a skills lab setting. This is then followed by practice on a pig's trotter or simulated skin. Pigs' trotters come closest to real skin, provided they are obtained fresh and used on the same day, but they have little subcutaneous fat, unlike in humans. In countries where pigs' trotters cannot be used (e.g. for religious reasons) simulated synthetic skin could be used. This is far more expensive and far less realistic. Ideally one should practise suturing under the supervision of a tutor who has the experience and the expertise to teach. It is also useful to get a senior colleague to observe and advise, when suturing real patients for the first time. Most doctors would have done this in their undergraduate or early postgraduate career. However, nurses and nurse practitioners who undertake training must be supervised by experienced peers or general practitioners, at least on the first few occasions.

In certain settings the suturing can be delegated to an experienced trained nurse. Unless the nurse has been adequately trained in the diagnosis of wounds and injuries, it is advisable for the doctor to assess the patient prior to delegating the suturing task to the nurse. It must be remembered that every 'superficial wound' or 'minor cut' is potentially a deep wound, and the size of the wound is no reflection of the depth of the wound or the extent of the injury. Assessment and diagnosis is a clinical skill, while suturing superficial wounds is essentially a technical skill.

Reflections

- Are you familiar with the sutures that you would normally use and stock in the surgery?

- Are you confident and competent in suturing?

- Are you familiar with the clinical anatomy of, and important superficial structures in, the various anatomical areas of the human body?

It is useful to acquire skills in the following suturing techniques:

- Simple interrupted suture
- Vertical mattress suture
- Subcuticular suture
- Buried suture
- Gillies three-point suture.

Correction of dog-ears is another very important and useful skill to learn. In the following paragraphs, some of the important points to be aware of when undertaking these procedures are discussed.

Simple interrupted sutures

This is the basic and most commonly used suturing technique. Your supervisor will show you how to handle the needle holder and where to hold the needle, with the jaw of the needle holder. Remember that the appropriate tools are as important as the technique! Choose the right type and size of instruments. It is the duty of the surgeon to brief the nurse, regarding the type of instruments that need to be sterilised for the particular procedure. It will be useful to have a protocol or checklist of instruments for the various procedures. It is important to think about any additional instruments you may need for the individual procedure, rather than regret not having the appropriate instrument after starting the operation. Communication with the nurse who will assist you is very important. Stitchcraft can only be learnt under supervision from an experienced person.

Points to note

- Appropriate handling of the needle holder and forceps.
- Appropriate holding of the needle.
- The wrist movements and appropriate entry of the inserting tip of the needle (at right angles to the skin surface).
- Adequate 'bite' of tissue and optimal distance (usually about 5 mm) from the edge of the wound.
- Exit at the appropriate distance from the second edge.
- Adequate number of loops and throws for a surgical knot (double loop in first throw, single loop in second throw), adjusting the knot on the side of the wound and tightening just enough to slightly evert the edges. Remember to 'square the knot'.
- Using an extra throw of double loop, with monofilament materials, to ensure that the knot does not slip.
- When placing epidermal sutures, a pear- or egg-shaped bite is required, taking a greater bite of dermis than epidermis, which optimises apposition of edges with a tinge of eversion (Figure 9.3).

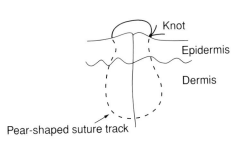

Figure 9.3 Pear-shaped suture tract.

Some pitfalls to be avoided

Problem	Possible outcome
Sutures too loose	Wound opens, poor scar and possible sepsis
Sutures too tight	Does not allow for wound oedema; sutures may cut through
Sutures too far apart	Potential for wound opening up
Sutures too close	Potential for greater scarring/marking
Edges inverted	Tendency to dimple/poor cosmesis
Edges overlapping	Poor scarring. Can be rectified at the time of suturing
Dog-ear redundancy of wound end	Ugly scar with redundant skin. Can be repaired primarily at closure
Knot tails too long	Can get stuck together. More difficult for nurse to remove

Buried sutures

Sometimes deep wounds are best closed by placing subcutaneous, absorbable deep sutures which help to obliterate dead space, and bring together the open wound sufficiently to help the surgeon to do the skin suturing without tension. They also help to prevent wound dehiscence after the epidermal sutures have been removed. In vertical buried sutures, the knot is 'buried' at the deeper plane. The insertion of the needle starts in the deepest plane, and the needle moves upwards, exiting at the wound via the more superficial dermal plane, followed by re-entry on the other side of the wound via the dermal plane, passing vertically downwards and exiting via the deepest plane, parallel to the entry at the opposite side of the wound. The knot is then tied, and is buried in the deepest plane. This often brings the skin almost into apposition, only requiring epidermal skin suturing which can be done without tension. Depending on the site, one could even use strips like Steri-strip® or Leuko-strip® to appose the skin edges together. Alternatively, subcuticular suturing technique could be used to bring the skin edges together (Figure 9.4).

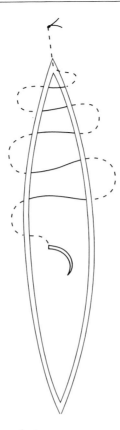

Figure 9.4 Subcuticular suturing technique.

Dog-ear repair

The bunching of skin at the end of the wound occurs when suturing circular skin defects or elliptical defects where the angle of the ends is over 30°. Closure of the wounds 'by halves' results in a dog-ear at both ends, while suturing from one end to the other leads to redundant skin at only one end. Many techniques of repairing a dog-ear have been described.[1] One such technique is shown in Figure 9.5.

Vertical mattress suture

The vertical mattress stitch is one of the best ways of ensuring that the apposition of the edges of the skin is slightly everted. It is also used

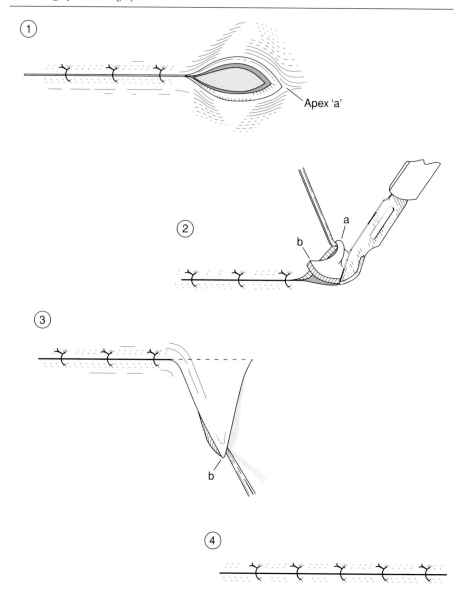

Figure 9.5 Dog-ear repair.

for apposition of deep wounds, without buried sutures. It can be used to obliterate dead space. It also helps in reducing the tension at the site of suturing and, if properly placed, the superficial, epidermal bite will have least tension. It takes time and is more technical than a simple suture. It is important to ensure that the bites are at equal distances from the edge (Figure 9.6).

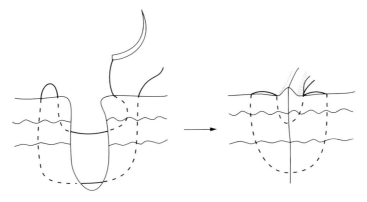

Figure 9.6 Vertical mattress suturing.

Subcuticular suturing

This needs greater technical skill, but has the advantage of avoiding multiple puncture marks, which may last for a long time, and is therefore cosmetically superior to placing simple interrupted sutures. But it is vital to ensure that the wound is not closed under tension. Often, buried sutures in the deeper layers reduce the tension and enable better placement of subcuticular sutures without tension. Straight or curved needles can be used (*see* Figure 9.4).

Three-point suture

This corner stitch of the tip of a triangular wound helps to reduce the chances of the tip necrosing (Figure 9.7).

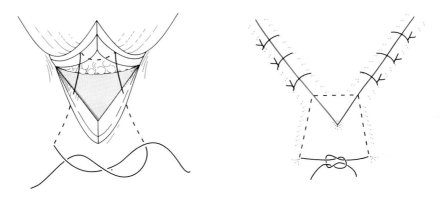

Figure 9.7 Gillies three-point suture technique.

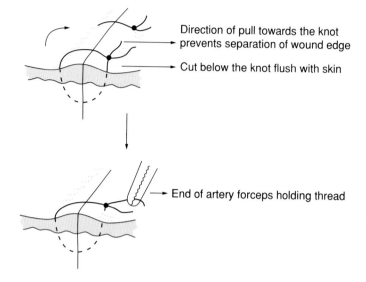

Direction of pull towards the knot
prevents separation of wound edge

Cut below the knot flush with skin

End of artery forceps holding thread

Figure 9.8 Removing a suture.

Removal of sutures

This important area is often delegated to the practice nurse. It is important to ensure that the nurse understands and is trained to remove sutures in the appropriate way, at the right time. It is better to remove sutures a little later than earlier, the latter leading to wound dehiscence. Counselling the patient regarding what he can and should not do is important. Occasionally reinforcing the wound with skin strips for a further period may be required, if there is doubt over the wound strength. The direction in which the thread is pulled may determine the probability of the wound opening up. Holding the knot thread with gentle traction, cutting the suture *below the knot*, and gently pulling along the plane of the skin *towards* the side of the knot, reduces the separating influence of the traction. If the wound is not fully healed at the expected time, it may be wiser to leave at least alternate sutures for a further period (Figure 9.8). Steri-strips® are a useful adjunct.

References

1   Borges AF. Dog-ear repair. *Plast Reconst Surg.* 1982; **69**(4): 707–13.

10

Opening and closing

A minor surgery is one performed on someone else!

Overview

- Pre-operative assessment and counselling of patient:
  - on the day of the operation
  - pre-operative procedure
  - positioning of the patient and the area to be operated
  - adjusting the lighting
  - hand washing/hand disinfection/surgical scrubbing
  - transient and resident flora
  - preparation of the skin.
- Access (subcutaneous and deeper lesions):
  - planning the incision – Langer's lines versus relaxed skin tension lines (RSTLs)
  - vertical incision, including the full skin thickness
  - see what you do – avoid 'blind' dissection
  - dissect in anatomical planes
  - avoid damage to neuro-vascular structures
  - secure adequate haemostasis.
- Assess:
  - macroscopic confirmation of clinical diagnosis
  - the best way to remove the lesion without damage to surrounding structures.
- Action.

- Exit:
  - avoid dead space
  - ensure haemostasis
  - avoid tension when closing the wound
  - precise coaptation of the edges.

Pre-operative assessment and counselling

Unless there be correct thought, there cannot be any action,
And when there is correct thought, right action will follow.

Reach a decision *with* the patient to operate on the lesion after assessing the site and nature of the lesion. **Always** explain what you intend to do and the usual and possible outcomes, especially cosmetic effects and other complications. Remember the five 'A's' (age, associated illness, allergies, anticoagulants and anxiety) when assessing the patient.

Remember

- Counsel the patient on complications and cosmetic effects (e.g. scar and dyspigmentation) and *document* it.

- 'Informed consent' means the patient must be able to make a fully *informed* decision – taking into account both usual and unusual outcomes.

- Evidence that the patient has been informed adequately, in the form of *legible documentation* in the patient's notes, is very important, irrespective of getting written consent.

- It is now recommended that the patient is given time to think about your counselling and advice about the procedure, before electing to have the intervention. It is not advisable to counsel and then operate on an individual on the same day for a routine procedure, especially skin lesions.

On the day of the operation

Ensure that the practice nurse is fully aware of the procedures you intend to do, and the instruments you require. Do not forget to mention the type and size of the sutures you intend to use. This makes it easier for the nurse to prepare the nurse's trolley. It is good practice to have a checklist of equipment required for the procedures you do. This is very useful for the practice nurse, who must ensure that you have all the equipment sterilised and available for the operations.

Pre-operative procedure

Make sure that the patient *understands* the procedure you intend to carry out, and the possible outcomes. Explore any concerns the patient may have. Get written consent if possible. It is useful to document this by including a statement to that effect in the consent form; or writing it *legibly* in the patient's notes.

Positioning the patient and the part to be operated

The patient must be comfortable. The part to be operated needs to be positioned appropriately, e.g. side arm board if needed, for surgery on the upper limb.

Adjust the lighting

This is best done by the surgeon before hand washing.

Hand washing and 'scrubbing'

> *Soap and water and common sense are the best disinfectants.*
> Sir William Osler (1849–1919)

Types of skin flora

The two types of skin flora are *transient* and *resident flora*. Micro-organisms deposited or acquired from the inanimate environment, including furniture and other surfaces, and from other patients are known as transients. They do not multiply on the skin, and can be removed by frequent hand washing or disinfection. Transients include organisms that may cause cross-infection, such as *Staphylococcus aureus*, *Escherichia coli*, *Pseudomonas aeruginosa*, *Proteus* species, *Klebsiella* species and *Salmonella* species.

Resident flora do not usually cause cross-infection. Residents are mainly Gram-positive coagulase-positive cocci (e.g. *Staphylococcus epidermidis* or other staphylococci), aerobic and anaerobic diphtheroids. They can cause infection by introduction during invasive procedures such as surgery or insertion of intravenous lines. The residents colonise the hair follicles and deeper layers and crevices of the skin.

Three procedures need to be considered:

- hand washing
- hand disinfection
- surgical scrub.

Hand washing

Hand washing is the most important way of preventing cross-infection. Unless hand washing is done in a systematic way, some of the areas will be missed. The areas commonly missed by poor technique are shown in Figure 10.1. These include the fingertips and nail fringes, web spaces and palmar creases.

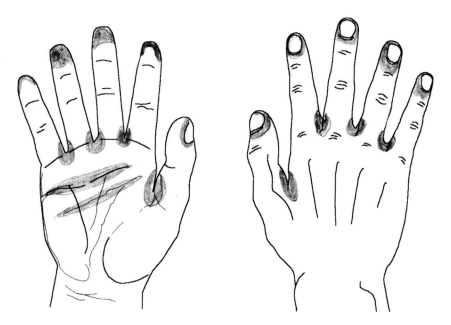

Figure 10.1 Areas likely to be missed (shaded) if hand washing is not done in a systematic way.

Hand washing using bar or liquid soap removes dirt, grit and most of the transient flora. It does not remove the resident flora. A systematic thorough wash with a cosmetically acceptable soap removes most of the transient organisms which are responsible for cross-infection. This is adequate for all routine patient examinations. If done thoroughly, it could remove 99% of the transient flora.

Hand disinfection

An antiseptic soap or detergent is used for the removal or destruction of all or most transient organisms. A residual effect is preferable. The common antiseptics used are chlorhexidine, povidone-iodine or triclosan. A thorough hand disinfection over 15–30 seconds is very effective in disinfecting the hands. Of the three antiseptics, chlorhexidine (4% w/v) has the least sensitising effect, and is less allergenic than povidone-iodine.

Surgical scrub

Remove rings, wrist watches, bracelets or any other jewellery before scrubbing. Surgical scrub using antiseptics is used to remove or destroy almost all the transient micro-organisms *and also to remove the majority of the detachable superficial resident micro-organisms*. A prolonged effect is required. The nails need to be brushed and antiseptic applied to the hands and forearms for a contact time of a minimum of 2 minutes, using a systematic technique of scrubbing. The scrubbing should extend proximally to mid-forearm. Since a high proportion of surgical gloves are punctured, depending on the nature and duration of the procedure, it is important to do a surgical scrub in order to ensure that most of the transients and the superficial residents are removed or destroyed. Ensure that the entire hand is scrubbed properly in a systematic way.[1] Use of a brush to clean the nails is important for the first scrub, but *not* for subsequent procedures. In fact, repeated use of the brush could damage the skin and encourage microbial proliferation and surfacing of the deeper residents. Hands should be dried using sterile towels before donning the gloves.

Chlorhexidine and triclosan have a sustained residual activity, which discourages the multiplication of organisms that are deposited subsequently on the skin. The application of an alcoholic hand rub destroys the transients and superficial residents on the surface of the skin. This is even more effective than aqueous antiseptics, but must be applied after hand cleansing.

Some definitions

- Sterilisation: destruction or removal of all forms of life (including spores).
- Disinfection: destruction or removal of all vegetative bacteria, viruses and fungi, but not bacterial or fungal spores.
- Antisepsis: disinfection of living tissues.
- Decontamination: removal of pathogenic micro-organisms so that surfaces are safe to handle.

Reflections

The four important elements in hand disinfection and scrubbing are:

- the *type* of antiseptic used

- the *technique* of cleansing

- the *duration* of scrubbing

- the *extent* (area) of scrubbing.

Preparation of the skin

Solutions used for skin preparation are a personal choice. Remember that povidone-iodine is better for clostridial spores, but that its allergenicity is higher than that of chlorhexidine. The duration of contact is important.

Planning the incision

This is very important and determines the type and extent of scar. *Remember that relaxed skin tension lines are **not** the same as Langer's lines.* Consider whether primary skin closure can be achieved without tension. Mark the skin if necessary. Special pre-sterilised skin markers, which will not induce tattooing, are available commercially, but they are not cheap. The aim should be to place the incision clear of the lesion by at least 1 mm, and preferably 2 mm if there is doubt about the pathology of the lesion.

Langer's lines and relaxed skin tension lines

> *Error flies from mouth to mouth, from pen to pen, and to destroy it takes ages.*
>
> Voltaire (1694–1778)

Many surgeons and authors confuse the differences between Langer's lines as originally described by Langer, and the crease lines, which are relaxed skin tension lines (RSTLs). The first documented observation on skin papillae and skin lines in the West, was by Cloquet in 1816. Dupuytren made the first documented observation of the distortion of skin wounds after stabs in 1834. On the 26 April 1861, Professor Langer presented a paper at the Proceedings of the Society of Natural History of Vienna 'On the Anatomy and Physiology of the Skin'. The first part, on 'The Cleavability of the Cutis', was based on his study of cadavers.[2] Kraissl,[3] in his seminal paper, was the first to critically appraise Langer's work and clarify the distinction between Langer's lines and crease lines or wrinkle lines. Langer's lines, for example, are at right angles to the creases across joints. Incisions along Langer's lines over joints may lead to hypertrophic scars and contractures!

- Crease lines or wrinkle lines are related to the underlying muscles and joints. They run at right angles to the long axis of the muscles.
- These lines become more prominent with ageing skin, due to the loss of elasticity, lengthening of the collagen fibres and damage to the skin by sunlight.
- To ensure minimal scarring and maximal cosmesis, incisions should run *parallel to* or *within* crease lines or RSTLs.
- RSTLs can be determined by gently pinching the skin between the thumb and forefinger in two axes perpendicular to each other. Note the plane in which the skin wrinkles with greatest ease, and make the incision on or parallel to it.
- Relax the skin by movements of the joints close to the planned incision, before attempting to pinch.
- Another way of determining this is to make a circular incision around the lesion and excise it. Now observe that the open wound is not exactly circular, but oblong. This long axis is the RSTL. You will notice this if and when you do punch biopsies using the Stiefel or similar biopsy punch. In my experience, the scar and cosmesis are better with circular incisions for lesions that are very small (under about 7 mm in diameter). In larger lesions, circular incisions may lead to dog-ears that need to be rectified when closing.

- Remember that RSTLs in the anterior chest of a female are different from those in a male. They tend to be horizontal (transverse) over the breasts (Figures 10.2 and 10.3).

The simplest rule for making incisions in the most favourable direction is to follow the natural wrinkle lines.

JP Webster (1935)

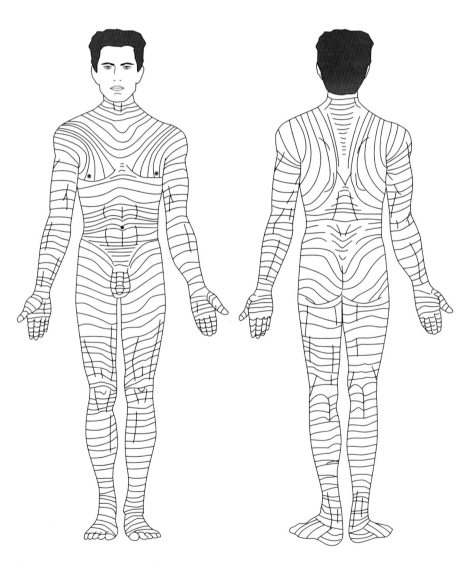

Figure 10.2 RSTLs on the front and back of a male.

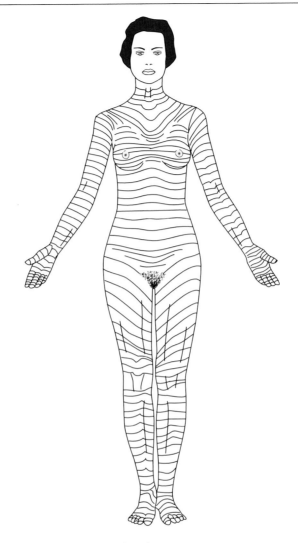

Figure 10.3 RSTLs on the front of a female.

Reflections

- Observe the wrinkle lines of the middle-aged and elderly people around you. Note the way the wrinkles are accentuated when the muscles contract. These lines are best observed during emotive expression (laughing, smiling, crying).

- If you operate on the face, it is important to have a selection of fine suture materials, and appropriate instruments to handle them. Analyse the RSTLs over the face to minimise scarring.

continued

continued

- Are you familiar with the anatomy of the face and the surface landmarks[4] for the identification of key anatomic structures of the face and neck?

- Where is the glabella?

- Where are the vermilion border and the philtrum?

- Where are the naso-labial line and the mental crease?

Access

Points to remember:

- vertical incision including the full skin thickness
- avoiding fish-tail edges in elliptical incisions
- see what you do; good light is important
- adequate haemostasis
- technique of soft-tissue dissection, and undermining if required.

In linear incisions, it is important to determine the length of the incision, which should allow adequate exposure. Remember the old aphorism:

Big mistakes are made through small holes!

It is advisable to have at least a 3 : 1 ratio of longitudinal to transverse axis of the fusiform or elliptical incision, to prevent dog-ears. Dog-ears are redundant aggregates of skin produced by the forced movement of tissues. The bunching up of the skin at the wound ends, when they are sutured, can be avoided if one is aware of the elasticity of the skin in the area to be operated and plans the elliptical incision appropriately. However, in very small lesions, one could make a circular incision around the circumference of the lesion and use dermal suturing techniques without dog-ears. It is good practice to have at least a 1 mm clearance around all cutaneous lesions that look clinically benign, and 2 mm around lesions where you are doubtful of the lesion. *Clinically malignant lesions are best referred, especially malignant melanomas.* The circular excision[5] is becoming increasingly popular for circular lesions as it minimises the removal of excessive normal skin on either side. Dog-ears are dealt with in the usual way.

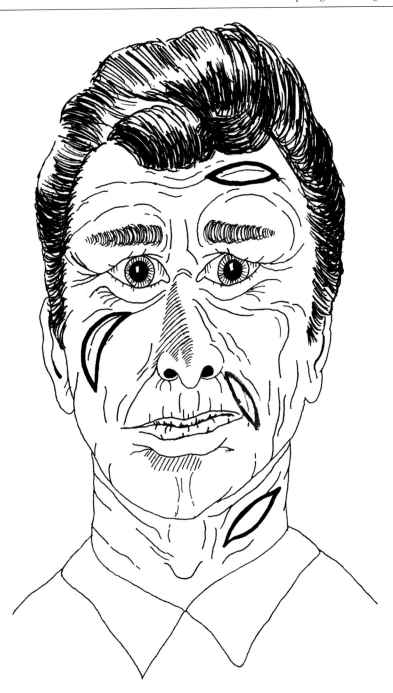

Figure 10.4 RSTLs on the face.

Soft-tissue dissection and undermining can be achieved using small, curved, blunt-nosed scissors. This instrument is invaluable in the excision of the majority of cutaneous and subcutaneous lesions excised by general practitioners.

In areas where there is little subcutaneous tissue, such as the face, one should take great care in undermining due to the high risk of damaging nerves and vessels. This can be avoided by injecting about 2–5 ml of normal saline for injection, subcutaneously immediately prior to the incision, after the local anaesthetic has been injected, in order to elevate cutaneous lesions. This technique reduces the risk of damage to underlying structures. However, if too much saline is used, there is a potential for distorting the anatomical planes.

Reflections

- Can you enumerate the uses of scissors in minor surgical procedures?

- Can you enumerate at least four ways of achieving haemostasis in minor surgery?

Assess

Points to remember:

- macroscopic confirmation of diagnosis
- does the appearance of the lesion confirm your clinical diagnosis? The final diagnosis will depend on the histology
- can the lesion be removed without damaging any significant vessels and nerves in its proximity?

Action

Points to remember:

- complete removal of the lesion without crushing the lesion while handling

- adequate haemostasis
- check that nothing has been left behind in deeper planes.

Complete macroscopic removal of all lesions is important. This is achieved by dissection in the appropriate planes. For example, cutaneous lesions will need dissection in the subcutaneous plane. Undermining, if required, is often done in the subcutaneous plane.

Exit

Points to remember:

- *avoid* dead space
- *adequate* haemostasis
- precise coaptation of the skin *without* any tension
- appropriate dressing and support.

The problem of potential dead space rarely arises in cutaneous surgery, as one hardly goes into deeper anatomical planes. But if the subcutaneous fatty layer is thick, the need to use a buried suture may arise to obliterate the dead space and bring the skin edges closer together, thereby reducing the tension on the epidermal sutures that are used for the final apposition of skin edges. A 4/0 or 3/0 absorbable suture material can be used for subcutaneous fat. Dead space can be avoided by undermining and placing deep sutures, or by closing the wound in layers.

Always ensure that there is no active bleeding before closing the wound. Pressure and patience usually easily control venous oozing. Active bleeders may need to be cauterised, or ideally electrocoagulated, after holding the vessel with a suitable artery forceps. For deeper wounds, subcutaneous interrupted, absorbable sutures, such as Vicryl®, could be used to reduce the chances of haematoma later, especially if a large lesion has been removed, leaving a potential dead space. Ensure that the contact dressing is sterile and preferably non-adherent.

Following a shave procedure, where the wound is oozing and will not be closed, chemical haemostasis can be achieved if pressure does not stop the ooze. Three solutions are often used.

- Aluminium chloride. Comes in aqueous and alcoholic solutions of varying strengths, 20–70%. The alcoholic solution is best avoided if electrosurgery or radiosurgery is used, due to the potential for igniting the wound. Aqueous aluminium chloride, 35%, is highly recommended as it is a very effective clear solution and does not cause staining or tattooing of the tissues. It has no effect on surrounding normal tissues.

- Ferric subsulphate, 20% (Monsel's solution). In the experience of some, Monsel's solution is more effective than aluminium chloride.[6] There is a small risk of tattooing.
- Silver nitrate. This is available as a stick or solution. It tends to cause scarring or tattooing quite often, and is slow to effect haemostasis after shave biopsies. Often used by hospital specialists on the cervix, and for granulomas.

It is worth remembering that the ultimate aim of wound closure is to bring together all the tissue layers that have been opened, and finally coaptation of the edges without tension, and mild eversion, which will lead to a neat scar.

Usually the dressing (depending on the site) keeps the wound clean and protects it until wound healing is well under way. The type of dressing used is more often a matter of choice by the surgeon or nurse, their preferences depending on the nature, cost and availability.

Post-operative advice

- Don't forget to inform the patient about what to expect in the early days.
- Advise or dispense analgesics for post-operative pain. Advise on posture, use of the affected part and return to work.
- Post-operative written instructions will be most useful for patients.
- Ensure that follow-up arrangements have been made, *before* the patient leaves the surgery.

Remember

- Always recapitulate the anatomy of the area on which you are going to operate.

- The patient and the surgeon must be relaxed.

- Ensure that all the instruments and equipment you need are available before starting.

- Send all specimens for histology.

- Follow up the patient and the histology.

References

1   Field EA, Jedynakiewicz NM and King CM. A practical gloving and hand-washing regimen for dental practice. *Br Dent J.* 1992; **172**: 111–13.

2   Langer K. On the anatomy and physiology of the skin: 1. The cleavability of the cutis. *Br J Plast Surg.* 1978; **31**: 3–8.

3   Kraissl CJ. The selection of appropriate lines for elective surgical incisions. *Plast Reconst Surg.* 1951; **8**: 1–28.

4   Bernstein G. Surface landmarks for the identification of key anatomic structures of the face and neck. *J Dermatol Surg Oncol.* 1986; **12**: 722–6.

5   Davis TS, Graham WP and Miller SH. The circular excision. *Ann Plast Surg.* 1980; **4**(1): 21–4.

6   Larson PO. Topical haemostatic agents for dermatologic surgery. *J Dermatol Surg Oncol.* 1988; **14**: 623–32.

11

Wound dressings and bandages

Overview

- Types of wound closure.
- Stages of wound healing.
- Primary contact dressings.

Wound closure

I dressed him and God healed him.

Ambroise Pare (1510–1590)

Wound closure is usually classified according to the time delay between an operative procedure and closure:

☺ primary wound closure
☺ delayed primary wound closure (after 4–5 days – closed by direct suture or skin graft)
☺ healing by secondary intention.

Primary wound closure is the object in almost all routine minor surgical procedures. As the majority of lesions removed in primary care are small (less than 1 cm), primary wound closure is the norm.

Delayed primary wound closure is performed in situations where primary wound closure may not be possible, due to oedema or excessive tension when apposing the edges, or when the wound is badly contaminated despite wound cleaning.

In healing by secondary intention, the wound is not closed and healing occurs by granulation. Although the mechanism of healing is the same, the duration of the various stages of healing varies.

Stages of wound healing

Acute inflammatory phase

Lasts 0–5 days. This commences within minutes of the injury of a surgical incision and usually lasts about 3 days. During this phase the fibrin clot is formed which helps to seal the apposed edges of the wound. The surgical incision leading to injury of the skin results in histamine and serotonin being liberated into the wound from vasodilatation and increased permeability of the vascular endothelium. This is the cause of postoperative wound oedema. If the sutures apposing the wound edges are too close to the edge of the wound and/or tied too tightly, they tend to cut through and early wound dehiscence is likely. Hence the importance of the suturing technique, which is both an art and a science, that has to be learned by practising under supervision. The white cells (leucocytes) and macrophages have an important role in ensuring the removal of dead tissue and bacteria. The neutrophil leucocytes mainly ingest the bacteria and facilitate the action of macrophages by the release of fibrinolytic and other proteolytic enzymes. Cleaning and removal of debris also occur during this phase.

The proliferative phase

Days 5–14. Granulation and vascularisation occur during this phase. The macrophages are also responsible for the neovascularisation that follows and play an important role in the formation and function of fibroblasts. During the proliferative phase which lasts about 14 days, the inflammation subsides. A rapid increase in wound strength occurs in this phase. *Epithelialisation* commences around 24 hours after the injury. The epithelial cells on the surface grow over the edge of the wound over the underlying dermis, and across the wound defect under the dried fibrin scab. In primary wound healing this process takes about 2–3 days.

The maturation or remodelling phase

Day 14 until complete wound healing. This can take up to a year. Although collagen levels peak around 3 weeks after an injury, the tensile strength of the scar keeps increasing gradually, over a year or so, although no more collagen is formed. The randomly orientated collagen fibrils gradually become orientated in the direction of maximal stress, resulting in a stronger scar. However, only about 75–80% of the normal tensile strength is achieved after recovery.

Wound dressings

He should bind with clean white cloth, for if they are not clean, harm results. He should also wash his hands before he treats anyone.
Heinrich von Pfolspeundt (1460)

Thomas defined a dressing as a material which, when applied to the surface of a wound, provides and maintains an environment in which healing can take place at the maximum rate.[1]

An *ideal dressing*[2] will provide the optimal milieu for the early healing of a wound. The dressing should:

☺ allow the wound to remain moist; a moist environment enables epithelial cell migration and enhances viability of these cells
☺ be vapour permeable, allowing gas exchange
☺ provide thermal insulation, since a warm environment is important for healing to occur
☺ be free from too much exudate or slough; an optimal amount of exudate is conducive to healing, as it contains nutrients and growth factors
☺ act as a barrier to micro-organisms or other particles/foreign bodies
☺ remain undisturbed until healing is well under way
☺ be non-adherent and easily removed, without traumatising the wound
☺ be non-toxic, non-allergenic and non-sensitising.

Types of wound dressings

Primary wound contact materials, usually used following primary skin closure, include the following.

Paraffin gauze dressings

PROPERTIES
- Low-adherent wound-contact material.
- Made from open-mesh cotton, viscose, rayon or gauze impregnated with white or yellow soft paraffin.
- Not highly absorbent.

USES
For low- to medium-exuding wounds, as in clean, superficial wounds, skin grafts or after partial phenolic matrixectomy for ingrowing toe-nails (IGTN).

EXAMPLES
- Jelonet® (Smith & Nephew).
- Paranet® (Vernon-Carus).
- Paratulle® (Seton).
- Unitulle® (Roussel).

Medicated tulle dressings, such as Bactigras®, are not indicated in most minor surgical procedures.

Low-adherent non-medicated primary contact dressing

PROPERTIES
- Provide protection.
- Made from different materials, such as cotton/acrylic fibre and knitted viscose.
- Not highly absorbent.
- Low adherence.
- Perforated dressings.

USES
Surgical wounds healing from primary closure and superficial wounds.

EXAMPLES
- Tricotex® (Smith & Nephew). Sterile knitted viscose dressing.
- N-A Dressing® (Johnson & Johnson). Sterile knitted viscose dressing.

- Mepore® (Molnlycke).
- Melolin® (Smith & Nephew).
- Release® (Johnson & Johnson).

Mepore®, Melolin® and Release® are absorbent, perforated plastic-film-faced dressings.

Semipermeable film dressings

PROPERTIES
- Polyurethane, transparent, adhesive-coated semipermeable films.
- Non-absorbent.
- Vapour permeable to varying degrees.
- Impermeable to water and micro-organisms.
- Retain the exudate at the wound surface, ensuring a moist environment.

USES
- Surgical wounds after primary closure, scalds, abrasions, superficial ulcers.
- May be used as a secondary dressing to hold an absorbent dressing in place.

EXAMPLES
- Bioclusive® (Johnson & Johnson).
- Opsite® (Smith & Nephew).
- Tegaderm® (3M).
- Cutifilm® (Beiersdorf). Cheaper than Tegaderm®.

In both Bioclusive® and Opsite®, the adhesive film is based on a piece of release paper that is divided into three parts. The central portion of the paper is removed and the film is applied on the sutured wound, before the two outer pieces of the backing paper are removed. In Tegaderm® the film is sandwiched between a sheet of release paper on the adhesive side and a thin card on the outer surface.

Medicated film dressings are usually not used in minor surgical wounds.

Secondary wound contact materials are *not* routinely used in minor surgery. Their main use is for absorption of large amounts of exudate, debridement and some have antibacterial action, in addition to protection. These include alginate dressings (e.g. Kaltostat®, Sorbsan®), deodorising dressings (e.g. Actisorb Plus®, Carbonet®), enzymatic debriding agents (e.g. Varidase®), foam dressings (e.g. Lyofoam®, Allevyn®), hydrocolloid dressings (e.g. Granuflex®, Tegasorb®) and hydrogel dressings (e.g. Intrasite® gel, Clearsite®).

Bandages

Bandages are used for one or more of the following purposes:

- to retain the primary or secondary dressing
- to provide support
- to provide protection
- to provide compression.

They can be classified into different types, depending on their nature:

- extensible bandages
- non-extensible bandages
- tubular bandages
- adhesive/cohesive bandages
- medicated paste bandages
- orthopaedic casting materials.

In minor surgery, the extensible bandages and the tubular bandages are used most often. The extensible bandages are classified into different groups depending on their conforming, supportive and compressive properties.

Type 1: *lightweight conforming stretch bandages*

Their main function is to retain dressings and they are usually made of lightweight elastomeric threads. They are not capable of much compression.

EXAMPLES
Polyamide and cellulose contour bandages such as:

- K-Band® (Parema). Cheaper than Kling® or Stayform®
- Easifix® (Smith & Nephew)
- Stayform® (Robinson)
- Slinky® (Seton)
- Kling® (Johnson & Johnson).

Type 2: *light support bandages*

Crepe bandages are an example of this type. They do not exert significant pressure.

Type 3: compression bandages

These bandages can provide light compression, medium compression, high compression and extra-high compression. Graded compression stockings used for the management of varicose veins belong to this type.

Surgical tape

Micropore® and Scanpor® are commonly used. Scanpor® is cheaper and as effective.

Swabs

Non-woven swabs are cheaper than woven swabs, and therefore more cost-effective.

Reflections

- What are the stages of wound healing?

- What are the features of an ideal dressing?

- What post-operative, primary contact dressings are used in your practice?

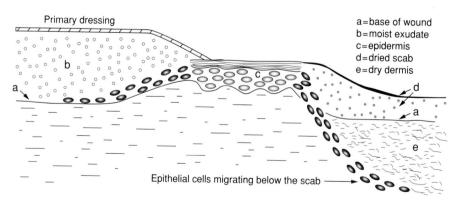

Primary dressing

a=base of wound
b=moist exudate
c=epidermis
d=dried scab
e=dry dermis

Epithelial cells migrating below the scab ⟶

Figure 11.1 Effect of moist environment on epithelial migration.

References

1   Thoms S. The role of foam dressings in wound management. In TD Turner, RJ Schmidt and KG Harding (eds) *Advances in Wound Management*. Chichester, John Wiley & Sons; 1986.

2   Turner TD. Hospital usage of absorbent dressings. *Pharm J*. 1979; **222**: 421–2.

Further reading

It is highly recommended that you look up the latest drug tariff and MIMS to check the relative prices, as prices may have changed since publication.

12

Ingrowing toe-nails

In the context of present day standards of nail surgery, many patients might be better off having the germinal matrix phenolised by a skilled chiropodist.

AW Fowler, *The Lancet* (1975)

Overview

- Prevalence and types of IGTN.
- Anatomy of the normal nail apparatus.
- Management of IGTN; prevention and treatment:
  - options for treatment
  - important points about phenolisation.

Prevalence and types

Ingrowing toe-nail (IGTN), or onychocryptosis, is very common in primary care. Although it could occur at any age, the majority occur after adolescence. The degree of involution of the lateral edge into the sulcus or nail groove seems to increase with age.

Boll[1] in 1945 documented the first known description of matrix phenolisation. He described three types of nails in three different age groups.

- Type 1: in young adults between 10 and 20 years. Normal contour nails. Lips and flaps are hypertrophied. Granulation tissue in nail groove.

- Type 2: seen in adults. Increased convexity. Lateral edges pressing firmly into nail groove, which is usually shallow.
- Type 3: nail plate is markedly curved and cutting into nail bed. Like type 1, this shows hypertrophy of the lips and granulation tissue is also marked.

The types of treatment recommended also differed.

Presentation

The anatomy of a big toe with the nail is shown in Figure 12.1. Most patients present with discomfort, pain or infection with granulation tissue, acute and chronic paronychia or associated fungal infection and nail deformity. Usual predisposing or aggravating factors include faulty technique of nail cutting, hyperhidrosis and pressure from footwear that is too tight, especially in schoolgoing adolescents and female patients.

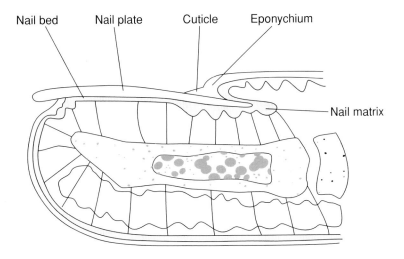

Figure 12.1 Sagittal anatomy of nail apparatus.

Management

Prevention

A 'toe watch' programme is needed. Foot hygiene is important, especially in diabetics. Toe-nails must be cut across horizontally, and the corners should not be cut obliquely but straight. Narrow shoes should be avoided.

Treatment

This depends on the degree and type of IGTN, and the presence or absence of complications. Consider the five 'A's too (age, associated illness, allergies, anticoagulant/aspirin therapy and anxiety). Purulent, 'smelly' toes are better managed by toe hygiene and antibiotics initially. Although there is no hard evidence for the use of antibiotics, a 1-week course of an antibiotic effective against staphylococci seems sensible. Further delay in definitive treatment is unnecessary since partial excision of the nail matrix and/or phenolisation with or without removal of the granulation tissue helps the inflammation to subside earlier.

Options of treatment

- Partial excision of nail (recurrence rate around 75% at 1 year).
- Total nail removal.
- Partial excision of nail *and* partial chemical (phenolic) matrixectomy.
- Partial excison of nail *and* partial surgical matrixectomy (by cutting and curetting).
- Partial excision of nail *and* partial radiosurgical matrixectomy.
- Total nail removal and phenolic matrixectomy.
- Total nail removal and radiosurgical matrixectomy.
- Total nail removal and total surgical matrixectomy (Zadik's[2] procedure).
- Partial or total nail removal with radio wave matrixectomy.[3]

Zadik's procedure is hardly ever done in primary care, as the results of phenolic matrixectomy are equally good, and recovery is quicker and less painful.

Phenolic partial matrixectomy

- Position the patient and foot on the operating table.
- Adjust the light.
- Anaesthetise the big toe, using lignocaine 1% by giving a ring block. Ensure that the entire toe is anaesthetised adequately.
- Use cut end of a glove digit to place around the toe as far proximally as possible, and roll the distal cut end of the rubber proximally, which will help to reduce the vascularity of the toe.
- Pull the ring of tourniquet and place an artery forceps.
- Proceed with skin preparation, using an appropriate solution (povidone-iodine or chlorhexidine).
- Check that the anaesthetic is working!
- Insert a nail plate elevator, under the area of nail you plan to excise, and separate the adhesion between the nail plate and the nail bed. The elevator must be inserted far enough towards the proximal end of the nail plate.
- Cut the nail, longitudinally from the distal end, extending proximally under the proximal nail fold.
- Grip the portion of the nail to be removed with a small Kocher forceps or a large straight artery forceps and by gentle pronation/supination movement of the wrist, separate the segment, and remove it.
- Place the nail segment with its root over the nail bed and assess the proximal extent of the root behind the proximal nail fold. Mark it if necessary. This gives you an idea about the distance you have to push the cotton stick with phenol, to destroy the lateral horn of the germinal matrix.
- Having ensured that the cotton stick dipped in phenol is not dripping, insert the cotton stick into the angle of the proximal and lateral nail fold and push the cotton stick up to the proximal end of the nail root area.
- Ensure that no phenol drips onto normal skin. Smearing petroleum jelly or paraffin on the surrounding skin may reduce the possibility of phenolic burns.
- 'Rub' the stick into the germinal matrix until it takes on a bluish-white hue (about 2 minutes).
- Use a dry cotton stick to remove any free phenol that may remain.
- Do not forget to remove the tourniquet now or after the dressing is applied! I use paraffin gauze followed by a swab, and tubinette dressing secured by an adhesive tape (Micropore®/Scanpor®).

Advise the patient about driving, standing and analgesics if needed for the next few days. The dressings are changed at 3 days and thereafter weekly by the nurse or patient, until the oozing stops. The patient can be taught to do the dressing after bathing. It usually takes about 3–6 weeks for the wound to be healed and dry.

Reflections

- Are you familiar with the anatomy of the human nail?

- Can you identify the matrix area, lunula, eponychium, cuticle, proximal nail fold (PNF), dorsal, intermediate and ventral nail plate, and nail bed?

- If you are not familiar, it is worth revising from an anatomy, chiropody, dermatology or orthopaedic textbook.

- Do you have access to all the instruments required for treating an IGTN?

SOME IMPORTANT POINTS ABOUT PHENOLISATION

- Phenolisation is best done under *tourniquet* in a dry field.
- If you don't have a flat rubber band (stationery type), a cut rubber glove finger, with the distal end cut too, is rolled over the big toe from distal to proximal, and clamped with a mosquito forceps (which will remind you to remove the tourniquet after phenolisation). The tourniquet is put on *after* the ring block.
- **Never** use adrenaline with the local anaesthetic for digits. Plain lignocaine (1%) or 0.5% bupivacaine (which is longer acting) could be used. Remember to give adequate time for the anaesthetic to take effect. Equal volumes of both can also be used, to harness the benefit of longer-acting bupivacaine.
- Use *liquefied phenol 80%* (or 85%) w/w in water, prepared recently. (Your pharmacist will oblige.) It should be *colourless*.
- The phenol should be stored in a *brown glass bottle*, and kept away from direct sunlight – preferably in a cupboard beyond the reach of any children. Although a glass stopper is ideal, they are hard to come by, and a glass dropper and rubber top is adequate. Old light-exposed phenol changes to yellow, pink and even brown with time. However, there is no evidence that it is less effective. Although the colour may not change for many months, it is recommended that liquefied phenol is not used after a month or two. Shapiro[4] has noticed that some 2–3-year-old phenol supplies are clear and colourless.

- Orange-stick cotton swabs are convenient and efficient. Wet them with phenol, but they should not drip. *Phenol that drips onto normal skin will cause chemical burns.* Excess phenol can be blotted off by using a gauze swab, thereby preventing phenol from dripping out of the matrix and sulcus onto the normal skin.
- By laying the partially or completely excised nail plate with its root *over* the eponychium, one can fathom the length of proximal extension of the matrix. This gives an idea as to how far proximally the orange-stick needs to be pushed, in order to destroy the matrix chemically. There is no evidence to show that curetting in addition to proximo-lateral matrix phenolisation is superior to the latter alone.
- Varying *phenol contact time* has been used, from 30 seconds to 5 minutes. About 2 minutes is adequate. When the colour of the matrix changes to a light whitish-blue hue, it would suggest adequate contact time. Washing with alcohol (as traditionally done in the past) is not required. Once the phenol has been rubbed into the matrix cells it cannot be neutralised by alcohol. The use of alcohol is contrary to the object of the exercise.
- After phenolisation, the matrix area should be dried using cotton-tipped orange-sticks.

Non-adherent contact dressings and tubular gauze are used. Re-inspect after 2–3 days. The patient could be given the dressings thereafter for self-application after a bath. It is important to have clear follow-up plans. The patient should know when to seek nursing or medical opinion post-operatively. Written instructions to reinforce the verbal explanations and instructions will be most useful. This will include mobilisation, footwear, elevation, analgesics, work and when to seek help. Warn the patient that serous oozing may sometimes continue for up to a month. The latter is the main disadvantage of phenolic matrixectomy.

In the long term, recurrence is a possibility. This varies from 0% in a randomised retrospective survey of 30 patients by Siegle *et al.*[5] to 7% in a randomised control study of 54 treatments by Morkane.[6]

After removal of the nail partially or totally, the destruction of the germinal matrix is achieved by using one or more of the following methods:

- manual excision and/or curettage
- chemically, using phenol
- using thermal cautery
- cryosurgery
- radio waves (using an Ellman Surgitron or similar equipment).

In partial matrixectomy, the aim of treatment is to destroy the lateral horn of the germinal matrix on one side of the nail.

Radio wave technique

The use of radio wave electrodes to destroy the germinal matrix was initially reported by Kendall in 1988.[7] If you have a radiosurgical instrument such as the Ellman Surgitron, and there is no contraindication to the use of radiosurgery (pacemaker in the patient), a useful accessory to acquire is the matrixectomy set of electrodes. These are insulated and have an active end which is 2 mm or 4 mm wide. The 2 mm wide instrument is very useful for partial matrixectomy because it can be inserted into the angles. The proximal extent to which you insert the electrode can be assessed by replacing the excised nail plate and root over the nail bed and eponychium to note or mark the proximal extent to which the nail extends (Figure 12.2). The main advantage of radio wave ablation is that the prolonged oozing that often follows after phenol treatment is avoided.

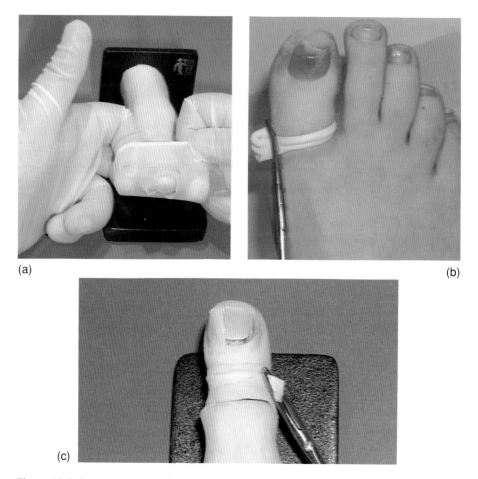

(a)

(b)

(c)

Figure 12.2 Ingrowing toe nail: (a) applying tourniquet (b) with tourniquet and clamp in place (c) nail placed over the nail bed to show proximal extent of germinal matrix.

Reflections

- Do you give written advice for IGTN and other procedures in your practice?

- Have you had any feedback from your patients, regarding the usefulness of the instructions?

- What is the important principle of partial or complete matrixectomy?

References

1   Boll OF. Surgical correction of ingrowing toe nails. *J Natl Assoc Chirop.* 1945; **35**(4): 8–9. Reprinted in *Br J Chirop.* 1974; **39**: 75.

2   Zadik FR. Obliteration of the nailbed of the great toe without shortening the terminal phalanx. *J Bone Jt Surg.* 1950; **32B**: 66–7.

3   Hettinger DF, Valinsky MS, Nuccio G and Lim R. Nail matrixectomies using radio wave technique. *J Am Pod Med Assoc.* 1991; **81**(6): 317–21.

4   Shapiro SL. Observations on the phenol technique of nail matrix eradication. *Curr Pod.* 1969; **18**(1): 18–21.

5   Siegle RJ and Harkness J. Phenol alcohol technique for permanent matrixectomy. *Arch Dermatol.* 1984; **120**(3): 348–50.

6   Morkane AJ, Robertson RW and Inglis GS. Segmental phenolisation of ingrowing toe nails: a randomised control study. *Br J Surg.* 1984; **71**(7): 526–7.

7   Kendall MW. Radiosurgery: an advanced technique for performing nail matrixectomies. *Pod Management.* 1988; **7**: 53.

Further reading

Dagnall JC. The history, development and current status of nail matrix phenolisation. *Chiropodist.* 1981; **September**: 315–24.

13

Sclerotherapy for varicose veins

Overview

- The three 'S's of varicose vein management.
- Indications/contraindications for sclerotherapy.
- Advantages and disadvantages of sclerotherapy.
- Types of sclerosants and mechanism of action.
- Method of injecting/post-injection management.

Introduction

This chapter deals only with the primary care issues that need to be considered in sclerotherapy. It is important to be aware of the anatomy and pathology of varicose veins. Useful resources are given at the end of this chapter, under Further reading. The next occasion you encounter a patient with varicose veins, take the opportunity to observe the anatomy carefully, and test for perforators, which can also be palpated. I assume you will do this, before reading any further.

Never ASS-U-ME anything. It makes an ASS (of) U and ME!!

A cynic

Sclerotherapy for varicose veins needs experience gained by *supervised training* with patients. Attending a practical course with practice on synthetic simulated varicose vein limbs can help you to attain some degree of competence and confidence. It will be more appropriate to practise under supervision by an experienced colleague.

Sapheno-femoral incompetence and perforator reflux can be detected using the hand-held Doppler, in primary care. But a more detailed and accurate assessment could be made with a colour vascular scan in secondary care.

Before you embark on sclerotherapy

- Do you know the anatomy of the long and short saphenous systems?
- Do you know the sites of the common perforators?
- How will you detect the sites of the perforator veins?
- How will you select patients for sclerotherapy?
- What are the contraindications?
- Which sclerosant will you use, and at what strength?
- What regime would you use for ambulatory compression sclerotherapy?
- What will the follow-up plans be?
- How will you counsel the patient before and after the procedure?

Varicose veins can be managed by three 'S's:

- support
- sclerotherapy
- surgery.

Support

Useful in early, small varicose veins, or if the other two treatments are not possible. It is also useful in pregnancy.

The *conservative management* of early varicose veins includes:

- weight reduction if indicated
- appropriate support by wearing graded compression tights or stockings
- increased physical activity, which helps the calf pump
- avoiding prolonged standing. Standing could be an occupational hazard. Advise patients to stand on their toes for a few seconds, periodically, if they have to stand for a long time.

Graded compression tights can be purchased in different colours. Numbers 8–12, depending on the size and pressure (low-pressure veins), of graded tights are very useful. Jonelle and Elbeo are very effective. Other 'support' tights are sold with 'lycra' in the material, but do *not* confer graded compression. Graduated compression hosiery, including below-knee 'socks' for men, are available on prescription. The choice of colours is limited, which is a disadvantage for the treatment of young adults.

The graded compression provided by the prescribable compression stockings can be classified into three classes:

- class 1 compression: mild support; compression at ankle = 14–17 mmHg
- class 2 compression: moderate support; compression at ankle = 18–24 mmHg
- class 3 compression: strong support; for gross varicies; compression at ankle = 25–35 mmHg.

When prescribing a graduated stocking, the following details should be written on the prescription:

- class of compression
- open or closed toe
- above or below knee
- quantity: single or a pair (in the UK, those eligible for prescription charges have to pay for two if a pair is ordered).

Sclerotherapy

Ensure that *emergency equipment* for resuscitation is available, before embarking on sclerotherapy. In addition, you should be competent in basic life support (BLS) skills, which should be updated periodically.

Indications for sclerotherapy

- Cosmetic.
- Aches and pains in the legs. Linear pain along veins or throbbing pain/ache over starbursts or angiectides.
- Nocturnal cramps.
- Oedema.
- Combinations of the above.

The majority of the patients consult for cosmetic reasons. The occurrence of aches and pains in the legs, especially with prolonged standing, is common. Some complain about nocturnal cramps, and swellings around the ankle, especially towards the evening. Some patients may complain of venous claudication – a bursting sensation on walking, relieved by elevation of the legs. This is common in the post-phlebitic limb.

Varicose veins with sapheno-femoral incompetence could lead to complications such as:

- dyspigmentation – especially hyperpigmentation
- superficial thrombophlebitis
- deep vein thrombosis (DVT)
- pruritus
- varicose eczema
- ulceration
- haermorrhage.

Although phlebologists would use sclerotherapy despite the presence of sapheno-femoral incompetence, recurrences are less likely with surgery.

Which patients?

From the context of primary care, patients who fulfil the following criteria will be suitable for sclerotherapy:

- ☺ absence of sapheno-femoral incompetence
- ☺ small and medium-sized varicose veins (less than 10 mm)
- ☺ early low-pressure veins
- ☺ symptomatic varicosities below mid-thigh level
- ☺ absence of a recent history of DVT
- ☺ residual varicosities and post-surgical recurrences, especially below knee.

The majority of the varicose veins seen in primary care, especially in females, are early, low-pressure veins and below the knee. These are suitable for compression ambulatory sclerotherapy.

Contraindications for sclerotherapy

- ☹ Sedentary patient who cannot ambulate for whatever reason.
- ☹ Obesity.

☹ Patients on oral contraceptives. It is preferable to switch to the progesterone-only pill for 1 month before and after.
☹ Recent DVT or acute superficial thrombophlebitis.
☹ Sapheno-femoral incompetence (relative contraindication).
☹ High-pressure veins.
☹ Pregnancy.
☹ Allergies.

Advantages of sclerotherapy

☺ Quick.
☺ Convenient.
☺ Patients do not need to take time off work.
☺ Avoidance of anaesthetic.
☺ Cheaper than secondary care treatment.
☺ More cosmetic.
☺ Increases the efficacy of the calf muscle pump.

Disadvantages of sclerotherapy

☹ Possibly higher recurrence rate if indications are not adhered to.
☹ Pigmentation problems.
☹ Skin necrosis.
☹ Allergic reactions.
☹ Vasovagal syncopy.

It must be remembered that ambulatory compression sclerotherapy has three elements to the treatment: ambulation, compression and sclerotherapy. The aim of sclerotherapy is to initiate a chemical thrombophlebitis in the superficial varicose veins, near the perforators, which causes a collapse of the superficial veins and secondary fibrosis, while improving the venous drainage via the deep veins, facilitated by the calf pump.

Some points about sclerotherapy

• Two sclerosants are available on the NHS drug tariff. They are sodium tetradecyl sulphate (STS or STD) and ethanolamine oleate. Another useful sclerosant, which is *not* available on the NHS, is polydocanol. It is supposed to have a lesser tendency to cause reactions and anaphylaxis.

- STD injection (fibro-vein) – 2 ml and 5 ml ampoules; 0.5%, 1% and 3% strengths. STD 0.5% is used for thread veins, spider veins and telangiectasias; 3% is used for larger-sized varicose veins. Ethanolamine oleate (5%) has a lesser tendency to affect skin pigmentation. It is available in 2 ml and 5 ml ampoules.
- Always counsel patients on outcomes and complications.
- The perforators can be identified clinically by palpation. Inject close to the perforators.
- Inject into the lumen of a short segment isolated between two fingers.
- Always aspirate a little blood to ensure that you are in the lumen, before injecting. Often the blood enters the syringe before aspirating.
- Do not inject more than four sites at a time, for larger veins. Don't use more than 1 ml of 3% STD at a time. Each site will not need more than 0.2 ml.
- Apply immediate compression with a dental pledget and Micropore®.
- Instruct the patients to walk for at least 30 minutes immediately after the injection/compression; and daily thereafter.
- Explain to the patient about avoiding crinkling of the compression hosiery.
- Depending on the size and pressure of the veins injected, continuous compression is maintained for about 2–3 weeks. The traditionally longer period of compression is unnecessary. Avoid injecting during hot weather, as it is uncomfortable for the patient to have continuous compression for weeks.
- Syncopy is a fairly common side-effect of sclerotherapy. Room temperature is important.
- **Never inject into an artery.**

Further reading

Bergan JJ and Goldman MP (eds) *Varicose Veins and Telangiectasias – Diagnosis and Treatment.* St. Louis, Missouri, Quality Medical Publishing; 1993.

Fegan G. *Varicose Veins.* London, William Heinemann Medical Books; 1967.

Goldman MP. *Sclerotherapy: Treatment of Varicose Veins and Telangiectatic Veins.* St. Louis, Missouri, Mosby Year Book; 1991.

14

Injections and aspirations of joints and soft tissues: Part 1

Overview

- Important issues: site, nature, surface anatomy, indications and contraindications.
- Common joint and soft-tissue problems.
- Indications and contraindications for steroid injections.
- Complications of steroid injections.
- Prevention of joint infections.
- Types of steroid injections.
- Types of needles used.
- Joint aspirations.
- Frequently asked questions.

Introduction

Injections and aspirations in primary care are easy and convenient to do. But you have to be certain about:

- the *site* of the lesion or problem

- the *nature* of the lesion or problem, i.e. be certain of the diagnosis
- the surface and deep *anatomy* of the site you are going to inject
- the indications and contraindications for injections.

Some of the joint and soft-tissue conditions for which injection of steroids, with or without local anaesthetic, is used are given in Figure 14.1. The list is not comprehensive.

Back to basics – remember

The six pairs of tissues you will deal with:

- skin and fascia

- vessels and nerves

- muscles and tendons

- ligaments and capsule

- synovium and bursae

- bones and joints.

When you look at a point on the surface of the body, where you intend to inject, always visualise the structures you will go through from skin to bone or joint. If you are not sure, it is worth looking at an atlas of anatomy or one of the multimedia programmes available for the PC (e.g. Bodyworks/3D skeleton).

Arthrocentesis (Greek, *arthros* = joint; *kentesis* = puncture) of joint fluid is done for diagnostic and therapeutic purposes. Cortisone was the first steroid to be used in a joint in 1950, after being first used for the treatment of rheumatoid arthritis in 1948.

Indications for steroid injections (see Figure 14.1)

Always try conservative measures first: give advice about things to avoid and things to do. The judicious use of NSAIDs, support, splints, orthoses, etc. often obviates the need for injections. The time to inject is when these measures fail.

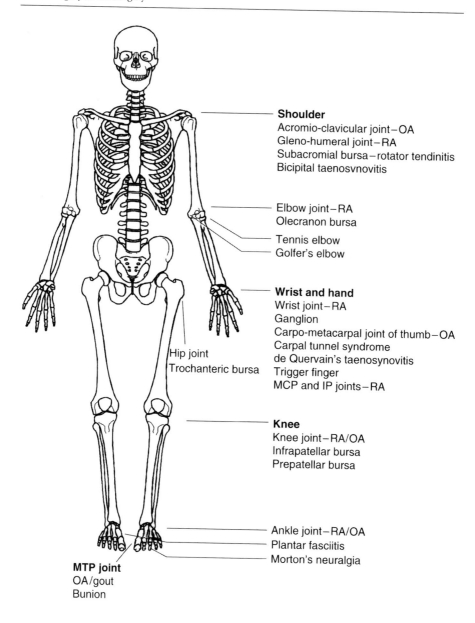

Shoulder
Acromio-clavicular joint – OA
Gleno-humeral joint – RA
Subacromial bursa – rotator tendinitis
Bicipital taenosvnovitis

Elbow joint – RA
Olecranon bursa

Tennis elbow
Golfer's elbow

Wrist and hand
Wrist joint – RA
Ganglion
Carpo-metacarpal joint of thumb – OA
Carpal tunnel syndrome
de Quervain's taenosynovitis
Trigger finger
MCP and IP joints – RA

Hip joint
Trochanteric bursa

Knee
Knee joint – RA/OA
Infrapatellar bursa
Prepatellar bursa

Ankle joint – RA/OA
Plantar fasciitis
Morton's neuralgia

MTP joint
OA/gout
Bunion

OA = Osteoarthritis
RA = Rheumatoid arthritis
MCP = Metacarpo-phalangeal
IP = Inter-phalangeal
MTP = Metatarso-phalangeal

Figure 14.1 Some of the joint and soft tissue conditions for which injection of steroids is used.

Contraindications to steroid injections

General

- Uncontrolled diabetes.
- Uncontrolled anticoagulant therapy.
- Known allergy to steroids (very, very rare).
- Septic skin (septic eczema/psoriasis).

Local

- Septic joint (as pirate).
- Overlying cellulitis.
- Local fracture (relative).

Complications

These are often due to poor selection of patients and poor technique.

Septic arthritis

This is the potential complication. It is extremely rare if proper aseptic technique is used. It is more common when injecting diabetics, especially those patients who are poorly controlled. It is more likely to be due to haematogenous infection rather than direct inoculation of skin bacteria into the joint.[1]

Haemarthrosis

This is caused by going through blood vessels. It is more likely in those with bleeding disorders (e.g. haemophiliacs) or in inadequately controlled patients on anticoagulants.

Sepsis could be prevented by

- Meticulous aseptic ('no-touch') technique.
- Alcohol (Mediswab®) is adequate for skin disinfection. Contact for 30 seconds removes most of the transient flora. A contact time of at least 2 minutes is important for an effect on superficial resident flora.
- Not removing the needle from the sheath until you are about to aspirate the steroid from the vial. Remove the 'lid' of the vial just before aspirating, and use Mediswab® to clean it. The rule is minimum exposure of sterile 'parts' to the atmosphere.
- Using disposable single-use syringes and needles.
- Using single-dose ampoules, when using lignocaine. (It is wise to avoid multidose vials.)
- Avoiding injection when the patient has cutaneous sepsis elsewhere or uncontrolled diabetes or bleeding disorders.

Which steroid?

The three commonly used steroids are:

1 hydrocortisone acetate (25 mg/ml)
2 methylprednisolone acetate (40 mg/ml) (Depo-Medrone® with or without lidocaine)
3 triamcinolone hexacetonide (20 mg/ml) (Lederspan®).

The potency and duration of action increase from (1) to (3). Depo-Medrone® with or without lidocaine (lignocaine) is the most convenient and most frequently used steroid in general practice.

Depo-Medrone® is available in 1 ml, 2 ml and 3 ml vials. The latter are more often used for relapse of rheumatoid arthritis, especially with severe polyarthritis. A stock of 1 ml and 2 ml vials is useful for general practice.

Depo-Medrone® with lidocaine (containing 10 mg of lignocaine hydrochloride) is available in 1 ml and 2 ml vials. The 1 ml vials come in boxes of 10 (Depo-Medrone® with or without lidocaine). The 2 ml vials come in single boxes.

The shelf-life of plain Depo-Medrone® is very much longer than that of Depo-Medrone® *with* lidocaine. This has implications for stock-keeping, depending on the usage.

Injection

This is best learnt by practising on simulated models, by attending a course. Follow up by doing some injections under supervision.

Needles commonly used

Colour	Gauge	Length	Bore
Orange	25G	16 mm/⅝″	0.5 mm
Blue	23G	25 mm/1″	0.6 mm
Green	21G	40 mm/1.5″	0.8 mm
White	19G	40 mm/1.5″	1.1 mm

The majority of the joints and soft tissue could be accessed with a blue, 23G needle for injecting steroids. Superficial, small joints could be accessed with an orange needle, but since the bore is narrow, the possibility of squirting methylprednisolone while injecting should be borne in mind.

Remember

Wider the bore of the needle, greater the pain!

Always be certain about the exact *site* of the pain and *nature* of the lesion. When assessing the shoulder, exclude referred or projected pain in the shoulder region. Pain originating from the shoulder does not radiate beyond the elbow. When testing individual or groups of muscles always test active, resisted and passive movements. If movement against resistance causes pain, it implies that the site of the problem is in the muscle involved.

Back to basics

Remember Appley's rule about examining any joint:

Look, feel, move

i.e. *inspect*, especially comparing both sides; *palpate*, especially for point tenderness; and *move* the joint. The latter includes active movements, attempted movements against resistance and passive movements.

Your clinical reasoning for deciding to inject will take into consideration the history, examination, the effect of the problem on the person's occupation, activities of daily living and the therapeutic response to other conservative options.

Remember

Point tenderness is the most important physical sign to elicit when determining the site of the lesion or problem. Localised tenderness excludes referred pain.

Injection with steroids is more useful in rheumatoid arthritis than in osteoarthritis. The accuracy of placement of the steroid injections has been in doubt. In one secondary care study from Nottingham[2] only half the placements were intra-articular. The experience of the doctor was not significant. Accurate injection was associated with successful aspiration of synovial fluids in the larger joints. This study also showed that the accuracy of the placement, even in the larger commonly injected joints such as the shoulder and knee, was only about 50%.

A further study, from Dublin,[3] comparing the accuracy of steroid placement with clinical outcome in patients with shoulder symptoms, showed that the accuracy of steroid placement significantly affected clinical outcome for certain ranges of movement, but not for pain.

Frequency of injections

It is recommended that one does *not inject more than three times a year, into large weight-bearing joints.*[4] This is due to the potential for more cartilage damage with frequent injections and possibility of steroid arthropathy from overuse after injection, which may worsen the arthrosis. In general, clinicians prefer a 6–12 week waiting period between injections for weight-bearing joints. Because of concerns for systemic absorption and adrenal suppression, most physicians advise injecting *no more than three major joints in a month*. Always reflect on *why* there was no clinical response to the first injection. Assuming that your needle placement was correct, was the diagnosis correct?

Repetition of injection is usually avoided for about 4–8 weeks for soft tissues and other joints. These clinical practices are more experience based than evidence based.

Joint aspirations

The purpose of joint aspiration is either for diagnostic or therapeutic reasons. Often it could be for both diagnosis and treatment.

Joint effusions

Effusions could be clear, as in rheumatoid arthritis and osteoarthritis, or cloudy or turbid, as in acute septic arthritis, gout or pseudogout. Haemarthrosis could be due to traumatic injury or anticoagulation therapy. The main indication for aspiration is for diagnostic reasons. However, large effusions cause impairment of function and pain. Aspiration is therapeutic under these circumstances.

Remember

- All joint aspirates should be sent for microscopy and culture.

- All turbid aspirates should be sent for urgent Gram stain and culture.

Frequently asked questions

Q. Do you have to wear sterile gloves when you inject joints?

A. Sterile gloves are not essential, but it is good practice to adhere to aseptic technique when injecting or aspirating joints. Wearing gloves is essential, if there is a possibility of exposure to the patient's body fluids. It is important to wear gloves if you are aspirating joints.

Q. Is it necessary to give a local anaesthetic before aspirating a joint?

A. Not required, due to the pain of injecting a local anaesthetic and the necessity to change barrels.

Q. How often can you inject steroids into joints?

A. Most rheumatologists and orthopaedists feel that a second injection, if indicated, should be given only after 4–8 weeks. It is also recommended that weight-bearing joints are not injected more than 3–4 times in a year.

Q. How many joints can we inject in one sitting with the patient?

A. It is advisable not to inject more than three large joints in a month. The type of steroid and the dosage also seem to have a bearing. When using long-acting steroids such as methylprednisolone for rheumatoid polyarthritis, I do not inject more than one large weight-bearing joint and two other non-weight-bearing joints. I do not exceed a maximum dose of 120 mg of methylprednisolone (Depo-Medrone®).

Q. Which steroid is most useful for injections?

A. Of the three commonly used steroids (hydrocortisone, methylprednisolone and triamcinolone), hydrocortisone is the shortest acting, while triamcinolone is the longest-acting drug. The duration of the response is inversely proportional to the solubility of the product in water. My personal preference is methylprednisolone, which is available as a 'plain' preparation or combined with lignocaine in the same vial (Depo-Medrone® + lidocaine).

Q. Is there an advantage in using multi-dose vials?

A. Multi-dose vials obviate the need for breaking ampoules every time you inject a person. However, there is a potential risk of cross-infection. Hence the recommendation to use single-dose vials in primary care.

Q. What are the more common adverse effects of intra-articular injection of steroids?

A. Vasovagal syncopy, not uncommon. Facial flushing, usually comes on within a few hours and can last for a few days.

References

1   Von Essen R and Savolainen HA. Bacterial infection following intra-articular injection. A brief review. *Scand J Rheumatol.* 1989; **18**: 7–12.

2   Jones A, Regan M, Ledingham J, Pattrick M, Manhire A and Doherty M. Importance of placement of intra-articular steroid injections. *BMJ.* 1993; **307**: 1329–30.

3   Eustace JA, Brophy DP, Gibney RP, Bresnihan B and Fitzgerald O. Comparison of the accuracy of steroid placement with clinical outcomes in patients with shoulder symptoms. *Ann Rheum Dis.* 1997; **56**(1): 59–63.

4   Zuckerman J, Meislin R and Rothberg M. Injections for joint and soft tissue disorders: When and how to use them. *Geriatrics.* 1990; **45**: 45.

Further reading

Dixon AStJ and Emery P. *Local Injection Therapy in Rheumatic Diseases.* Basle, Eular Publishers; 1994.

Silver T. *Joint and Soft Tissue Injection: injecting with confidence* (2e). Oxford, Radcliffe Medical Press; 1998.

15

Injections and aspirations of joints and soft tissues: Part 2

Shoulder pain

Shoulder pain is a *symptom* of articular (glenohumeral joint, acromio-clavicular joint), periarticular (subacromial bursa, bicipital tendinitis, rotator cuff tendinitis, adhesive capsulitis) or referred pain from the neck, lungs, heart or diaphragm.

Remember

If the patient can point to the site of pain with one finger *and* you can elicit localised point tenderness, it is *not* referred pain. The lesion is local – articular or periarticular.

Common shoulder pathology includes:

- glenohumeral arthritis (rheumatoid and osteoarthritis)
- acromioclavicular arthritis (as above, repetitive strain; for example clay-pigeon shooting)
- subacromial bursitis (often rheumatoid or from injury)

- rotator cuff tendinitis, especially supraspinatus tendinitis (painful arc with active movement, passive movement not restricted)
- adhesive capsulitis ('frozen shoulder')[1]
- bicipital tendinitis/taenosynovitis.

Remember

A trivial injury in an elderly person, leading to a *sudden loss* of active shoulder abduction, is due to a significant acute rotator cuff tear, which needs *emergency* orthopaedic referral. If repaired early the results are good.

Listen to the patient, he is crying out the diagnosis!

Attributed to Osler

Acromioclavicular joint

Pain induced in the joint by extreme movement of the upper limb, by moving the hand over the opposite shoulder, together with localised point tenderness over the joint suggests A/C joint pathology. Alternatively, the upper limb, which is held in the anatomical position, is pulled and adducted, behind the back, while the examiner who is standing behind the patient is palpating the acromioclavicular joint. The joint is easily palpated in most patients. It is difficult to inject more than 0.25–0.5 ml of steroid into this joint. I use a blue needle.

Subacromial bursa

Easy to access, by directing the needle below the acromion. If you are not confident in injecting the glenohumeral joint, bearing in mind that the subacromial bursa is often connected to the glenohumeral joint, injecting into this bursa will also benefit the glenohumeral joint. Injecting into this bursa is usually indicated for rotator cuff lesions, including supraspinatus tendinitis.

Glenohumeral joint

Can be approached anteriorly, using the coracoid process as a landmark, or posteriorly using the angle of the acromion as a landmark. My personal preference is for the posterior approach using a blue needle, or a longer green needle if I have to go through a greater muscle bulk. Enter with the needle about 1 cm or a thumb's width below the angle of the acromion, directing the needle along the axis formed between the thumb over the acromial angle and the index or middle finger over the coracoid process, when standing behind the patient. Frozen shoulder is a Dupuytren's-like disease, appearing from a fibrous contracture of the rotator interval and coracohumeral ligament of the shoulder joint.

Sheath of the bicipital tendon (bicipital tendinitis)

Palpate the bicipital groove first, by rotating the arm externally and internally, with the elbow flexed. In bicipital tendinitis, localised tenderness is felt just below the transverse ligament of the groove. Also resisted supination of the flexed elbow (at 90°) and held by the side of the trunk induces pain (Yergason's test). Flexing the shoulder against resistance with the elbow extended and held by the trunk induces pain (Speed's test). Do not inject against resistance, which may indicate that you are in the tendon, instead of the sheath.

Reflections

- Do you explain and counsel patients before injections?

- Do you get verbal or written consent? Where do you record it?

- What post-injection instructions do you give your patients?

- When do you follow-up patients after injection treatment?

- How frequently will you repeat the injections?

Elbow pain

Radiohumeral joint

Effusions here are seen on the posterolateral aspect in rheumatoid arthritis. One could aspirate it first, swap syringes while keeping the needle in, and inject steroids at the same sitting.

Elbow joint

Best approached posteriorly, with the elbow flexed.

Olecranon bursa

Can be aspirated easily. Steroid could be injected at the same sitting or subsequently if there is a recurrence.

Tennis elbow

Dorsiflexion of the wrist against resistance induces pain. Localised tenderness is characteristic.

Always warn the patient about lipodystrophy and skin dyspigmentation. Like in other soft-tissue conditions, initial management should include NSAIDs with orthoses and advice on activities at work, sport and recreation.

Remember

Medico-legally, it is recommended that whenever the chance of a complication or side-effect is more than 2%, the patient should be informed and documentation made in the notes that the patient has been informed. However, rarer outcomes need to be discussed if they have important implications for the patient.

Golfer's elbow

Here the problem is at the origin of the long flexors, at the medial epicondyle of the humerus (medial epicondylitis). The *ulnar nerve* enters the forearm, posterior to the medial epicondyle. Do not forget to warn the patient about lipodystrophy and dyspigmentation.

Pain in the wrist/hand

Wrist joint

Easier to enter dorsally. Palpate for the radiocarpal joint, on the ulnar side of the tendon of the extensor pollicis longus (EPL). I usually palmar flex the hand while applying traction by pulling on the hand, while the elbow of the patient is steady on the table. This manoeuvre opens up the wrist joint.

Ganglion

These usually arise from the synovial sheath of the tendons or the synovial lining of the capsule of the joint. More common on the dorsum of the wrist. Need a wide-bore needle to aspirate, and they are often dispersed by puncturing. Make sure that the lump is not expansile or pulsatile before any needling! Injecting with steroids can delay if not prevent recurrence. Hyaluronidase, either with or without steroids, has also been used. The recurrence rate is lower when hyaluronidase is used. In a prospective randomised study of 35 patients, comparing the treatment of ganglia by aspiration under LA and either instillation of steroid alone or with the prior use of hyaluronidase, the cure rate was determined at a cut-off point of 2 years.[2] The cure rate with combined use of hyaluronidase and methylprednisolone was 89% (recurrence rate of 11%), compared to 57% when treated by aspiration and instillation of methylprednisolone alone. If they are surgically excised either under a general or local (especially extensor surface) anaesthetic, the recurrence rate is lower but comparable to the use of methylprednisolone and hyaluronidase (10–15%).

In a larger, prospective, African study[3] on 340 consecutive patients, intralesional injection of hyaluronidase followed by fine-needle aspiration of the joint to dryness, 95% were cured at 6 months. The 17 patients who had a recurrence within 6 months had a re-aspiration. Unfortunately the follow-up was only up to 6 months.

The carpometacarpal joint of the thumb

This joint between the trapezium and the first metacarpal bone is a saddle joint. This is felt easily via the anatomical snuffbox – dorsolaterally. It can be felt with the tip of the finger, while actively moving the thumb. Feel it on your self, *now*! While palpating with your left thumb, extend first and then oppose your right thumb towards the right little finger. You can feel your right saddle joint moving under the tip of your left thumb! You can use a blue needle, and inject about 0.25–0.5 ml of methyl-prednisolone with lidocaine into the joint. Osteoarthritis of this joint is common.

de Quervain's[a] tenosynovitis

Causally linked notoriously to RSI (repetitive strain injury) which is now known as WRULD (work-related upper limb disorder). Thickening and crepitus on movement of the tendons may or may not be felt. Finkelstein's test[b] is very useful in early diagnosis. Approach the sheath while tensing the skin between the index and middle finger of your left hand (if you are injecting with your right hand). When injecting into the sheath, you can often feel the steroid tracking along the sheath, with a feeling of fullness under your fingers.

Trigger finger

Usually the ring finger is involved. The nodule is often palpable in the region of the metacarpophalangeal joint, at the level of the distal palmar crease. The majority of patients will respond to one or two injections. The response to steroids is better if the history is of only a few months. Although the discomfort and triggering stops, the nodule often continues to be palpable. Surgical release gives permanent relief, if symptoms persist after two steroid injections.

---

[a] Fritz de Quervain described, in 1895, stenosing taenovaginitis of the sheaths of abductor pollicis longus and extensor pollicis brevis at the wrist. He was the son of a pastor in Switzerland. Succeeded Kocher as professor of surgery in Berne.
[b] Harry Finkelstein described, in 1930, pain in the radial border of the wrist on rapid ulnar deviation of the thumb clenched in the palm. Emeritus surgeon, Hospital for Joint Diseases in New York.

Interphalangeal joints (proximal interphalangeal/distal interphalangeal)

Inject 0.25–0.5 ml of methylprednisolone with an orange needle or blue needle. Approach dorsolaterally.

Carpal tunnel syndrome

Try to determine the cause, if any. If bilateral, I usually inject one hand at a time. This median nerve entrapment syndrome at the wrist can present with pain (especially nocturnal pain), sensory disturbance, motor weakness and sometimes autonomic disturbance. Daytime pain is often seen if the wrists are used in flexion or repetitive tasks. Autonomic dysfunction is not rare, since 805 of the sympathetic fibres to the hand are contained in the median nerve. Hyperhidrosis, skin temperature changes, erythema and discoloration or diffuse hypersensitivity to touch have been described. Chronic compression leads to interference with the use of the hand for activities of daily living. Permanent sensory loss or impairment, with permanent weakness and wasting, can occur if the carpal tunnel is not decompressed surgically. This could lead to permanent impairment of hand function. It is a relatively simple procedure that could be carried out under local anaesthesia in most patients.

Of the many causes of carpal tunnel syndrome, rheumatoid arthritis and diabetes are two important causes. Any condition that causes overcrowding of the carpal tunnel, with pressure on the median nerve, causes symptoms.

Before you read any further, it is worth familiarising yourself with the anatomy of the carpal tunnel, the landmarks and the structures going through the carpal tunnel. Where is the ulnar tunnel? What is the canal of Guyon?

Back to basics

- The transverse carpal ligament extends laterally to the tubercle of the scaphoid, tubercle of the trapezium. Medially it is attached to the pisiform and hook of the hamate.

- Can you locate the palmaris longus and flexor carpi radialis in your hand? Oppose your thumb to the little finger with the

continued

continued

wrist slightly flexed. While keeping the pressure of your thumb against the little finger, gradually apply increasing pressure at the level of the distal wrist crease, medial to the insertion of the palmaris longus, with the thumb of the opposite hand. What do you see? See footnote for the answer![c]

• The other important landmark is the distal wrist crease.

Phalen's forced wrist flexion test[d] is the most sensitive test, and is positive in more than 80% of cases. Tinel's sign[e] is elicited by tapping the volar surface of the wrist at the distal crease or applying firm pressure, which triggers the sensory disturbance seen in carpal tunnel syndrome.

There are various approaches to the carpal tunnel. I approach the tunnel, medial to the palmaris longus, at the level of the distal wrist crease, via the fat pad, with a blue needle at an angle of about 45° to the skin. You can feel the 'give' after you have gone through the transverse carpal ligament. The reason for this approach is because it is very rare for any branches of the median nerve to take off from the medial side of the nerve. The sensory and recurrent motor branches usually come off the radial side of the median nerve. The recurrent motor branch usually comes off distal to the carpal tunnel, near the base of the thenar muscles; rarely it could arise proximal to the carpal tunnel, but radially.

One could argue that if you go into the nerve you will know, due to the pain inflicted along the distribution of the median nerve. You could then withdraw the needle a little and then inject without resistance. What would *you* do?!

There have been case reports of median nerve injection injuries.[4,5,6] Kasten[7] has suggested an even further medial approach, using the pisiform as a landmark, directing the needle distally and medially, aiming at the middle of the tunnel, going dorsally. A 1.5″ 25G needle is used, and pushed up to the hub of the needle. At this depth, when the hub is at the level of the skin, the tip will be dorsal to the median nerve.

I use a blue needle (23G, 1″) and 40 mg of methylprednisolone and lidocaine (1 ml vial). The patients are grateful for the immediate relief of paraesthesiae, which is worse than temporary numbness! But explain to the patient that it may be more painful the first night. I ask them to take

[c] You will see a bulge of fat pad. Approaching the carpal tunnel via this fat pad, medial to the palmaris longus, is less painful, and there is a lesser chance of damaging the median nerve, as you are going medial to it.
[d] George S Phalen described this in 1951 (*JAMA* 145: 1128). Phalen was an orthopaedic surgeon from Dallas, Texas. He worked at the Cleveland Clinic, Ohio.
[e] Jules Tinel described this in 1915.

analgesics for the first night, and I tell them that it will take a few days for the discomfort to go, and make them keep a diary and bring it for the follow-up appointment in 2–3 weeks. This gives them something to do! I advise them to avoid overuse for 24–48 hours. Hence I tend to do most of my minor surgeries on Fridays!

Remember the golden rule:

Do unto others as you would have them do unto you!

Reflections

- When do you follow up a patient after an injection/aspiration?

- What are the advantages of following up a patient after an injection?

- When will you refer a patient for surgical decompression of the carpal tunnel?

Summary

Carpal tunnel syndrome is common and important. If you are sure of the diagnosis, having excluded other possibilities, and conservative treatment with splint/NSAIDs/advice do not help, it is worth injecting. Ultrasound treatment has been used for short-term symptom relief.[8] However, if you are considering referral for ultrasound, the time is appropriate for surgical decompression. *Whenever you are thinking of repeating an injection, reconsider the diagnosis. This applies to any injection therapy.* Any evidence of thenar wasting or definite sensory loss impairment is an indication for surgical decompression as soon as possible. Steroid injection is useful to relieve symptoms even in these patients, while they await the surgical decompression.

Remember

- If there is *thenar wasting*, however slight, and/or objective sensory impairment or loss, surgical decompression should be done *as soon as possible*. Motor wasting and weakness hardly ever recover if delayed too long. You could inject while the patient awaits decompression.

continued

continued

- Conservative methods of treatment and injections help to relieve symptoms in the early stages, or while the patient awaits surgical decompression.

- If steroid injection therapy is used, always follow up the patient at periodic intervals, for recurrence of symptoms or objective signs.

- If the patient's symptoms are not significantly improved with the first injection, review your diagnosis and reassess the patient before repeating the injection.

- If there is a relapse or recurrence after the second injection despite lack of objective motor or sensory signs, consider referral for further investigations, such as nerve-conduction studies.

- The majority of carpal tunnel syndromes in younger patients will need surgical decompression.

Hip region

Hip joint

You will need at least a 2–2.5″ needle. The anterolateral and lateral approaches to the joint require positioning of the limb, and if you have not been trained to do this, these are best avoided. The greater trochanter is the important landmark. I use 80 mg of methylprednisolone with lidocaine.

Trochanteric bursa

Trochanteric bursitis is easily diagnosed. The patient will point, with one finger, at the greater trochanter area as the site of the pain. Patients point to the groin, anteriorly and more medially when the pain originates from the hip joint. You can elicit tenderness over the greater trochanter. Adducting the lower limb helps to locate the greater trochanter in more obese patients. Always 'pull before you push' the steroids. I use 80 mg of methylprednisolone with lidocaine.

Ischial bursitis

Occurs over the ischial tuberosity.

Adductor enthesopathies

Adductor enthesopathies of the thigh muscles (especially the adductor longus) in sportsmen and those doing aerobics is not uncommon. The diagnosis is made by asking the patient to point with one finger, eliciting localised tenderness, and stretching the origin by passive abduction triggers the pain or makes it worse.

Meralgia paraesthetica

The landmark here is the anterior superior iliac spine. This is an entrapment neuropathy of the lateral cutaneous nerve of the thigh as it penetrates the fascia of the upper thigh, about 4″ below the anterior superior iliac spine. Pressure here, followed by flexing the thigh, results in triggering the symptoms or exacerbating the paraesthesia and numbness. Sensory blunting of the anterolateral aspect of the thigh can be demonstrated if the entrapment is severe. I use a blue needle and inject 40 mg of methylprednisolone and lidocaine. Inducing numbness in the cutaneous distribution of the nerve indicates appropriate placement of the needle. Symptom relief can last from months to years. If it recurs early and there is sensory blunting, it may be wise to decompress surgically.

Knee

Knee joint

Can be approached laterally or medially. I use 80 mg of methylprednisolone with lidocaine (2 ml single vials). If I aspirate, I use a green needle and, provided the aspirate is not turbid, I swap syringes, leaving the needle in, and inject 80 mg of the above steroid. I usually provide Tubigrip® or crepe bandage for 48 hours, depending on the reason for injection, and advise the patient to 'rest' the joint for at least 48 hours, and restrict their ambulation to activities of daily living for a further week. They are reviewed at a fortnight.

Prepatellar bursitis (housemaid's knee)

This was an occupational hazard prior to the advent of carpets and hoovers!

Infrapatellar bursitis (clergyman's knee)

Anatomically there is a superficial bursa, anterior to the patellar tendon which is most commonly involved. The deep infrapatellar bursa is posterior to the patellar tendon.

Bursitis in front of the knee and the back of the elbow (olecranon bursitis) are usually from repetitive friction injury, often leading to thickening of the overlying skin also. They may be inflamed, but not infected.

Knee pain, like shoulder pain, could arise from articular and periarticular causes and be referred pain from the hip, especially in children. Careful palpation is the most useful tool for assessing knee pain.

Reflections

- Are you familiar with the anatomy of the tricompartmental knee joint?

- Do you know how to test the integrity of the collateral and cruciate ligaments?

- What is McMurray's test?

- How will you diagnose meniscal lesions clinically?

- Do you know how Baker's cyst, Osgood–Schlatter's disease and chondromalacia patellae present?

- What is Sinding Larsen's disease?[f]

- What are the bursae around the knee joint?

---

[f] Osteochondritis of the lower pole of the patella. The Norwegian surgeon described it in 1921.

Ankle joint/foot

Approached anteromedially. I usually go between the medial malleolus and tibialis anterior tendon, by palpating the tibiotalar joint space. The needle is directed posterolaterally. I use 40 mg of methylprednisolone with lidocaine via a blue needle.

First MTP joint

Indication: gout/osteoarthritis usually. Inject 0.5 ml of methylprednisolone plus lidocaine, via an orange or blue needle.

Plantar fasciitis

Determine whether mainly medial or lateral plantar fascia is involved. I approach it from the medial or lateral side, rather than through the sole.

Morton's neuralgia[g]

This is quite painful, and often caused by a neuroma. The patient often describes a burning pain between the third and fourth toes. Sometimes it is described as shooting pains. When it is between the third and fourth toes, it is worth exploring and excising the neuroma. Injection could be used while the patient is awaiting surgery.

Reflections

- Apley's aphorism of 'look, feel and move' helps you to examine systematically.

- In the case of the limbs, always compare with the opposite side.

continued

[g] Thomas George Morton (1835–1903): Neuroma of plantar digital nerve causing Morton's metatarsalgia, D1876. He was an orthopaedic, general and eye surgeon! Founder of the Philadelphia Orthopedic Hospital.

continued

- Remember that all three movements, i.e. active movements, passive movements and passive resisted movements, play an important role in the clinical examination.

- Localised tenderness is an important and useful physical sign.

- The majority of the joint and soft-tissue injections could be done with the blue needle (23G, 25 mm/1″, 0.6 mm bore).

- Steroid injections could be repeated after 2–3 months. But always reconsider your original diagnosis!

- Knowing when to refer is as important a skill as knowing how to inject!

- In rheumatoid arthritis, multiple small joints can be injected. I usually do not inject more than one large weight-bearing joint in one sitting, and do not exceed 120 mg of methylprednisolone in an adult. Intrasynovial steroids injected into two or more joints may induce hypopituitary–adrenal axis suppression for 2–7 days.[9]

- It would be advisable to rest, with mobility restricted to activities within the house, for about 2 days after injecting a weight-bearing joint. Currently there is no hard evidence regarding the duration of rest or limitation of activity.

- Intra–articular steroids also have a systemic effect. In polyarthritis, injecting the more inflamed joints results in benefit to all other joints.

- Always consider conservative management (e.g. NSAIDs/ orthoses /advice on work ergonomics/modification or avoidance of sports and recreational activities) before injecting.

Frequently asked questions

Q. How effective are the various modalities of treatment for shoulder complaints?

A. In general, for shoulder girdle disorders, manipulation may be superior, and for synovial disorders steroid injections seem to be the preferred method.[10] However, as a general practitioner, you may employ more than one modality at a time or at different times.

Q. Is resting the joint and patient necessary after intra-articular injection of steroids for rheumatoid arthritis?

A. Resting weight-bearing joints after injection seems to prolong the benefit of intra-articular steroid injections. In a study by Neustadt[11] a regime of post-injection 'prescribed rest', consisting of 3 days of bed rest followed by 3 weeks of limited ambulation using aids (crutches or cane), did prolong the therapeutic effect. A more recent study from Norwich[12] suggests that 24 hours of post-injection rest results in a significant prolongation of the clinical response and may reduce the need for frequent steroid injections.

Q. Are there any studies on the efficacy of common interventions for shoulder pain?

A. A recent review[13] of randomised controlled trials of interventions for painful shoulder highlighted the problems with selection criteria and outcome assessment. This stems from the lack of a standardised method of defining shoulder lesions. The authors concluded that there was little evidence to support or refute the efficacy of common interventions. The interventions included NSAIDs, intra-articular and subacromial glucocorticoid injections, oral steroids, physiotherapy, manipulation under anaesthesia (MUA), hydrodilatation and surgery. What is your experience? Have you reviewed your cases over the past few years?

Q. Can trigger finger be cured by steroid injection?

A. In a prospective study[14] on 58 patients with 77 episodes of taeno-synovitis of the flexor tendons, which was resistant to rest, NSAIDs and/or splinting, it was found that injecting with long-acting steroids such as methylprednisolone or triamcinolone was effective in nearly 90% of patients who were followed up to an average of 4.6 years. The symptoms and signs resolved in 61% of patients after the first injections.

References

1   Bunker TD. Frozen shoulder: unravelling the enigma. *Ann RGS England.* 1997; **79**: 210–13.

2   Paul AS and Sochart DH. Improving the results of ganglion aspiration by the use of hyaluronidase. *J Hand Surg Br Vol.* 1997; **22**(2): 219–21.

3   Out AA. Wrist and hand ganglion treatment with hyaluronidase injection and fine needle aspiration: a tropical African perspective. *J RCS Edinburgh*. 1992; **37**(6): 405–7.

4   Frederick HA and Carter PR. Injection injuries to the median and ulnar nerves at the wrist. *J Hand Surg*. 1992; **17A**: 645–7.

5   McConnell JR and Bush DC. Intraneural steroid injection as a complication in the management of carpal tunnel syndrome. *Clin Orthop*. 1990; **250**: 181–4.

6   Linsky ME and Segal R. Median nerve injury from local steroid injection in carpal tunnel syndrome. *Neurosurgery*. 1990; **26**: 512–15.

7   Kasten SJ and Louis DS. Carpal tunnel syndrome: a case of median nerve injection injury and a safe and effective method for injecting the carpal tunnel. *J Family Practice*. 1996; **43**(1): 79–82.

8   Ebenbichler GR, Resch KL, Nicolakis P *et al*. Ultrasound treatment for treating the carpal tunnel syndrome: randomised 'sham' control-led trial. *BMJ*. 1998; **316**: 731–5.

9   Gray RG and Gottlieb N. Intra-articular steroids. An updated assessment. *Clin Orthop Rel Res*. 1983; **177**: 235–63.

10 Winters JC, Sobel JS, Groenier KH *et al*. Comparison of physiotherapy, manipulation, and corticosteroid injection for treating shoulder complaints in general practice: randomised, single blind study. *BMJ*. 1997; **314**: 1320–5.

11 Neustadt DH. Intra-articular steroid therapy. In: RW Moskowitz, DS Howell, H Mankin and V Goldberg (eds) *Textbook of Osteoarthritis*. Philadelphia, W.B.Saunders; 1983.

12 Chakravarty K, Pharoah PD and Scott DG. A randomized controlled study of post-injection rest following intra-articular steroid therapy for knee synovitis. *Br J Rheumatol*. 1994; **33**(5): 464–8.

13 Green S, Buchbinder R, Glazier R and Forbes A. Systematic review of randomised controlled trials of interventions for painful shoulder: selection criteria, outcome assessment, and efficacy. *BMJ*. 1998; **316**: 354–60.

14 Anderson B and Kaye S. Treatment of flexor tenosynovitis of the hand ('trigger finger') with corticosteroids. A prospective study of the response to local injection. *Arch Int Med*. 1991; **151**(1): 153–6.

Further reading

Dieppe P, Cooper C, Kirwan J and McGill N. *Arthritis and Rheumatism in Practice*. London, Gower Medical; 1991.

Doherty M, Haazleman BL *et al. Rheumatology: Examination and Injection Techniques*. London, W.B. Saunders; 1992.

Ferrari R, Cash J and Maddison P. *Rheumatology Guidebook*. Oxford, Bios Scientific Publications; 1996.

Martin SD and Martin TL. Shoulder pain: rotator cuff tendinopathy. *Hos Med.* 1997; **33**(12): 23–4, 26–30, 46.

16

Complications of minor surgery

An expert is a man who has made all the mistakes which can be made in a very narrow field.

Niels Bohr

A summary of the various *potential* complications is given below, awareness of which is very important and needs to be considered in pre-operative counselling of the patient. Inadequate communication could lead to litigation by the patient. However, this should not put you off from doing minor surgery. The majority of these complications are uncommon. It will be a useful exercise to look at the left column of each table, and reflect how you would prevent the complication, before reading the right column.

Injections and aspirations

Provided you adhere to aseptic principles and techniques, injections and aspirations are safe. Never use adrenaline for end-artery areas, such as the fingers and toes, the potential complication of gangrene is high.

Local anaesthetics

Complication	Prevention
Systemic toxicity	Choose the patient appropriately. 'Pull' before you 'push'. Do not inject into a blood vessel. Inject slowly. Stop if there are any early symptoms of toxicity
Allergy	Check about previous allergy to anaesthetic agents
Intraneural injection	Patient may feel shooting pain. Never inject against pressure. Withdraw needle and inject
Intrathecal injection (Depo-Medrone® + lidocaine)	Know your anatomy. Never attempt unless you have had training in epidural injections

Steroids

Steroids are injected into synovial joints and into peri-articular areas. They are relatively safe. Be familiar with the preparations you use.

Complication	Prevention
Systemic steroids	
Facial flushing	Dose related. Usually harmless
Adrenal suppression	Occurs with large doses
Local steroids	
Septic arthritis (intra-articular injection)	Strict aseptic technique. Avoid injecting a patient with uncontrolled diabetes. Never inject into a septic joint or when there is a possibility of pre-existing bacteraemia
Lipodystrophy (soft-tissue injection)	Can occur after one injection. Not dose related. Warn patient
Crystal-induced arthritic flare	Occurs with long-acting crystalline preparations. Self-limiting
Dyspigmentation (soft tissue/VV)	Cannot predict or prevent. Warn patient
Tendon rupture (intra-tendinous injection)	Never inject against resistance – but in bad rheumatoid arthritis the tendons are degenerated and could have little resistance. Anatomical knowledge and 'feel' of tissues is important

Sclerotherapy

Complication	Prevention
Systemic	
Vasovagal syncope (common)	Having the room at the right temperature and ventilation helps. Minimise patient anxiety by counselling and explaining the procedure beforehand. More common with higher concentration of sclerosant (e.g. 3% sodium tetradecyl sulphate [STD])
Anaphylaxis (very rare)	Check for any reactions with previous injections of sclerosant
Local	
Extravasation with skin necrosis	Accurate placement of needle. Use finer needles and magnification loupes for finer veins and telangiectasias
Dyspigmentation	Warn patient. More common with STD than ethanolamine oleate
Thrombophlebitis	Avoid injecting until at least 6 months after previous DVT or thrombophlebitis, or if there is marked ankle oedema
Nerve damage (VV of legs)	Revise anatomy and be aware of the important cutaneous nerves, especially when injecting the leg
Prostatis (injection of piles)	Accurate placement of the needle is vital
Impotence (injection of piles)	Accurate placement of the needle is vital

Cryotherapy

Be cautious when using cryotherapy over the face and digits.

Complication	Prevention
Blisters/ulcers/sepsis	Avoid too long a 'freeze' time. Avoid too many freeze–thaw cycles. Warn patients
Scarring – cosmetic effects	Warn patients. Meticulous technique
Dyspigmentation (often hypopigmentation)	Warn patients

continued overleaf

continued from previous page

Complication	Prevention
Nerve damage	Know the anatomy of the area
Tendon damage	Know the anatomy of the area
Vascular damage	Know the anatomy of the area
Nitrogen-gas tissue insufflation	Anecdotal cases described in the literature
Severe oedema	Can be reduced by topical steroid (clobetasol propionate) ointment or a few doses of systemic steroid
Hair loss	Avoid too long a 'freeze' time

Operative complications

Complication	Prevention
Nerve damage	Anatomical knowledge, good light, adequate exposure and bloodless field are important. 'See what you do'
Vascular damage	As above
Tendon damage	As above

Post-operative wound healing

Complication	Prevention
Dehiscence	Advice on movement of the area. Appropriate technique of suturing, appropriate suture materials and strength. Avoid sepsis
Inflammation	Select appropriate suture materials. Monofilament causes less reaction. Good technique. Avoid sepsis
Infection	Avoid sepsis. Skin disinfection, gentle handling of tissues and strict asepsis. Prophylactic antibiotics if indicated

continued

continued

Complication	Prevention
Cellulitis	As above
Abscess	As above
Discharge	As above
Haemorrhage	Appropriate haemostasis. Avoid dead space
Haematoma	As above
Scarring – stretched/ hypertrophic/keloid	Depends on ethnicity and site. Warn patient. Proper apposition of skin edges, without too much tension

ALWAYS counsel the patient on possible outcomes, including cosmesis and scarring.

It is very useful to give the patient a *handout* on post-operative instructions, especially regarding analgesia, and about early features of complications.

Action

Write a post-operative handout for the common procedures you do (e.g. steroid injections, removal of skin lesions, IGTN, cryotherapy of lesions).

Reflections

BS (Bachelor of Surgery) – stands for **B**leeding and **S**epsis, the two early complications of surgery, and **S**carring is the late complication!

17

Audit and quality issues

Statistics is like a bikini. What they reveal is suggestive, but what they conceal is vital!

Audit and peer review are integral to quality issues in healthcare. Quality of care should be integral to practice. The semantics of audit is described in Appendix A.

Marshall Marinker[1] aptly defined audit as:

the attempt to improve the quality of medical care by measuring the performance of those providing that care by considering the performance in relation to desired standards, and by improving on this performance.

Audit, peer review, significant event analysis and critical incident analysis are integral to the subject of quality assurance. Why look at quality issues? McIntyre and Popper have given succinct comment:

Efforts to improve performance must come from a desire for self-improvement, a desire based on an essentially ethical insight. Audit must not be a part of a disciplinary instrument; it must be a tool for learning by feedback.

Audit is a powerful tool for self-directed learning.

Possible audits in minor surgery include areas of the Donabedian triad: structure, process and outcome.

Structure

Includes:

- space and adequate treatment room/'theatre'
- instruments: basic set and others depending on the procedures you do
- equipment (including resuscitation equipment, steriliser, cryo and cautery equipment)
- drugs (local anaesthetics/resuscitation drugs/oxygen?)
- records: manual/computer; *minor surgery book*; consent/written instructions to patients.

Some components of structure are 'essential' (minimum requirement), while others could be 'desirable' and some 'ideal'. For example, the availability and accessibility of resuscitation drugs is essential before undertaking any form of minor surgical procedures in primary care.

Reflections

- How big is your treatment room?

- Is there adequate light and ventilation?

- Is the resuscitation equipment available, adequate and accessible?

- How do you keep your records? Is there a separate minor surgery book? What columns do you have in it? Who checks them?

- Where are resuscitation drugs kept? Are they accessible in an emergency?

Process

- Waiting times for minor surgery.
- Pre-operative explanation (e.g. keloid/depigmentation).
- Consent: when applicable.
- Operative notes: indication (pre-operative histology diagnosis if possible, or at least whether benign, suspicious or malignant)/anaesthetic/procedure/findings/closure/dressing.

- Histology of lesions: procedures for recording and transport of specimens/forms/recording in the minor surgery book/notes/computer.
- Follow-up of patient and histology: when, where and by whom?

Reflections

- What happens in *your* practice? Who removes the sutures? Is it the surgeon or the nurse?

- Have you watched the practice nurse remove sutures? Is the technique correct?

- Who inspects the wound? Is there a system for review by the surgeon?

- When does the surgeon follow up the patient? Does the surgeon check the post-operative histology? Is there a system to ensure that the histology reports are received and checked?

- Quality assessment will involve looking at all these issues.

Outcome

Areas that could be looked at include:

- complications: short term, e.g. haemorrhage, *infections*; and long term, e.g. keloids/stretched scars
- comparison of pre-operative histological diagnosis with post-operative histology report, to determine diagnostic accuracy; being able to document whether a lesion is benign, suspicious or malignant is perhaps a minimum standard
- completeness of excision: though not relevant for benign lesions, this becomes important when removing suspicious or malignant lesions
- patient satisfaction: cosmetic and functional; depends on patient's expectations
- surgeon's satisfaction: reviewing your results from *your* perspective and expectations is illuminating. Sometimes the surgeon may not be satisfied with a stretched scar or other outcome, contrary to the patient! This gives the opportunity to review and perhaps revise the practice in future, to improve outcome.

Audit is one of the activities that enables a reflective practitioner to gain insight into his needs. Abraham Maslow described the three stages of learning as:

1   from unconscious incompetence to conscious incompetence
2   from conscious incompetence to conscious competence
3   from conscious competence to unconscious competence.

It is the first stage that is vital. In order to improve we need to be aware of our incompetence. This is the most important 'gap' we need to 'mind'. Audit is one of the tools that enables us to cross that gap from unconscious ignorance to conscious ignorance, giving us the motivation to improve. Some of the other methods include self and peer review, significant event analysis, critical incident analysis, problems posed by our patients during daily consultations and correspondence from hospital specialists.

Reflections

- How can you prevent complications? What is the incidence of post-operative infections in your practice? Could it be reduced?

- Will you operate on malignant lesions? How do you liaise with the specialists?

- Do you explain to the patient about the procedure you intend to perform and the possible outcomes? How do you ensure that he or she understands what you said?

- Does your nurse assistant explain the procedure while the patient is being positioned?

Appendix B is an example of a minor surgery audit. Although audit is an important tool of quality assessment, it is not the only tool. Periodic review of practice, significant event analysis (e.g. complications) and critical incident analysis (e.g. mortality) are very useful learning tools.

Do not believe in anything simply because you have heard it.
Do not believe in traditions because they have been handed down for many generations.
Do not believe in anything because it is spoken and rumoured by many.
Do not believe in anything because it is found written in your books.
Do not believe in anything merely on the authority of your teachers and elders.

*But after observation and analysis, when you find that anything
agrees with reason
And is conducive to the good and benefit of one and all,
Then accept it and live up to it.*
Siddharta Gautama the Buddha in Kalama Sutta (*c.* 600 BC)

Reference

1   Marinker M (ed.) *Medical Audit and General Practice* (2e). London, BMA; 1995.

Further reading

Brown JS. *Minor Surgery – A Text and Atlas* (3e). London, Chapman & Hall; 1997.

Excellent reference book. Audit: pp. 141–2.

Bull MJV and Gardiner P. *Surgical Procedures in Primary Care*. Oxford, Oxford University Press; 1995.

Both the above books cover all aspects of minor surgery comprehensively.

European Resuscitation Council. *Guidelines for Resuscitation*. 1994.

'Guidelines for basic life support', pp. 3–10, is important.

Evans TR. *ABC of Resuscitation* (3e). London, BMA; 1996.

'Recognising a cardiac arrest and providing .basic life support', pp. 1–4, is important. This is a book for your practice library.

Grol R and Lawrence M. *Quality Improvement by Peer Review*, Oxford General Practice Series 32. Oxford, Oxford University Press; 1995.

Richard Grol has written much on the concept of peer review. The authors cover the whole concept of peer review, which is an important dimension of quality assurance. This book is well worth reading.

Irvine D and Irvine S (eds) *Making Sense of Audit* (2e). Oxford, Radcliffe Medical Press; 1997.

Explains the what, why and how of audit.

Marinker M (ed.) *Medical Audit and General Practice* (2e). London, BMA; 1995.

Excellent introduction. Chapters on principles and standards are a must!

Sodera VK. *Minor Surgery in Practice*. Cambridge, Cambridge University Press; 1994.

Written by a casualty surgeon, p. 47.

Reflections

Does your practice use the *King's Fund Organisational Audit*, which looks at the quality issues in organisation of services? One of the sections (*standard 21*) includes the organisational quality issues in minor surgery. It is a checklist of 53 criteria, indicating three categories of weighting: *essential practice*, *good practice* and *desirable practice*. It is comprehensive and covers the organisational issues in practices doing extended (intermediate) surgery. Some of the criteria are not relevant. For example, criteria 24–27 are about general anaesthesia, which is not used in minor surgery.

The man who can smile when things go wrong has thought of someone he can blame it on!

Arthur Bloch

Discovering the degree of imperfection motivates the pursuit of perfection which is the hallmark of excellence.

Appendix A 'Jargonology'

*'When I use a word,' Humpty Dumpty said, in a rather scornful tone,
'it means just what I choose it to mean – neither more nor less.'*
Alice in Wonderland (Lewis Carroll)

- **Audit**: the systematic *critical analysis* of the quality of care. Its purpose is to identify and implement opportunities for improvement and to further the professional performance of those auditing their work. It involves repeated review, change or improvement.
  - Medical audit: audit activities concerning the performance of doctors. Initiated by the doctors.

– Clinical audit: audit of any aspect of healthcare provided by the members of the practice team.

Sometimes the more measurable drives out the more important.

- **Criterion**: a clearly *definable* and precisely *measurable* element of care, where one can say whether it is present or absent.
- **Standard**: a practice-agreed *extent* to which a criterion is achieved.
- *Criteria and standards are integral to any audit.* If one is pedantic about semantics – an audit without criteria and standards is not an 'audit'.
- **Quality**: the *degree* of excellence possessed.
  - Maxwell's six components of quality:
    - (i)   access to services
    - (ii) relevance to need
    - (iii) effectiveness
    - (iv) equity
    - (v)   social acceptability
    - (vi) efficiency.
  - WHO's four components of quality:
    - (i)   performance (technical quality)
    - (ii) resource use (economical efficiency)
    - (iii) risk management
    - (iv) patient satisfaction.

In the discovery of imperfection lies the chance for processes to improve.

Berwick (1988)

- **Quality assessment** is the process of evaluating the current level of performance.
- **Quality improvement** involves assessment but also a process of change and improvement. This is achieved by comparing the measured performance in relation to desired standards, and improving on this performance.
- **Quality assurance** requires both quality assessment and quality improvement which must be repeatedly reviewed and, if necessary, revised in order to maintain good quality.
- **Clinical (practice) guidelines**: clinical guidelines are systematically developed statements which assist in decision making about appropriate healthcare for specific conditions, based on the best current evidence. Guidelines are usually external.

Man tends to treat all his opinions as principles.

Herbert Agar

- **Practice protocol**: clinical guidelines modified by the practice, by agreement, and adopted as a code of procedure.
- **Peer review**: the consideration of performance by colleagues within the same profession or group, having comparable skills and experience.
- Audit and peer review are two useful methods of evaluating the quality of care provided by the practice team, and are powerful tools for continuing medical education.
- **Evaluation**: the procedure of gathering information about part or all of an event or activity for the purpose of making judgements about merit or acceptability. The purpose is often to recognise quality or improve it.
- **Assessment**: the process of measuring an individual's knowledge, skills or attitudes.

Objectivity, in short, has the logical status of a myth: it builds up one sense of reality rather than others. It is a myth whose attainment and maintenance demands of its subjects a rigorous and continued asceticism ...

Michael Novak

Appendix B Example of an audit on minor surgery

Minor surgery audit, April 1993–March 1994

Aims

1   To determine the proportions of various procedures done in the year.
2   To determine the incidence of 'incomplete excisions' in specimens sent for histology.
3   To determine the accuracy of the pre-operative histological diagnosis, by comparing the post-operative histology of the lesions sent.

Criteria and standards

For (2), ideally the incidence of incomplete excisions should be nil, for all lesions. The standard for all 'suspicious lesions' should definitely be nil.

For (3), the accuracy of pre-operative histological diagnosis must be 100%. The acceptable standard was taken as 80%, due to the low numbers involved.

Method

- From the operations register, determine the coding and proportions.
- Check all excisions sent for histology by looking up the notes; and determine the numbers which had a correct pre-operative histological diagnosis.

Results

Total number of procedures = 55

Injections	=	24	= 43.64%
Aspirations	=	5	= 9.09%
Incision	=	1	= 1.82%
Excision	=	20	= 36.36%
Cautery	=	2	= 3.64%
Cryotherapy	=	0	= –
Others	=	3	= 5.45%

The 20 excised lesions were:
Benign fibro-epithelioma   = 5. Sent for histology = 4
Benign fibrous histiocytoma   = 4. One had a pre-operative diagnosis
   of non-pigmented, benign lesion
Seborrhoeic keratosis   = 1
IGTN   = 6
Benign intradermal
   naevocellular naevus   = 3
Sebaceous cyst   = 1

18

Answers to minor surgery pre-course questionnaire

	Q1	Q2	Q3	Q4	Q5	Q6	Q7	Q8	Q9	Q10	Q11	Q12	Q13	Q14	Q15	Q16	Q17	Q18	Q19	Q20
a	T	T	F	F	F	F	T	T	T	T	F	T	T	T	F	F	T	F	F	T	F
b	T	T	F	T	F	T	T	T	T	T	F	F	F	T	F	T	T	F	F	T	T
c	F	F	F	T	T	F	T	T	T	F	T	T	T	T	F	T	T	T	F	T	T
d	T	T	T	T	T	F	F	F	F	F	F	F	T	T	T	F	T	F	F	F	F
e	T	F	T	T	T	T	T	T	T	F	F	T	F	T	F	F	F	T	T	F

Comments

Q1(c)   Vasectomy is not one of the procedures that attracts a fee.

Q2(a)   This is important to remember!

   (c)   If you do only 12 procedures in a quarter, you can carry over two to be counted towards the next quarter. However, if you do more than 15 procedures, the excess *cannot* be carried over to the next quarter.

   (e)   Not mandatory for minor surgery.

Q3(a)   Glutaraldehyde soaking is required for 10 hours to sterilise.

   (b)   Boiling for 5 minutes will disinfect instruments, but will not kill the spores.

   (d)   121°C for 15 min or 134°C for 3 min.

Q4   **Always** avoid adrenaline in LA, for the digits, penis or nose.

Q5(d)   Under 1% in Wall's series: Wall DW. *The Medical Annual 1985: the year book of general practice*. Bristol, Wright; 1985: 74–84.

Q10(a) Three minutes is adequate when using pure phenol. Methylated spirit neutralises phenol. Either this or a dry cotton bud is inserted to mop up any phenol. Ensure that phenol does not come into contact with normal skin.

(b)   It is always advisable to exclude sepsis by urgent microscopy, Gram staining and culture, the latter taking days. The injection could be given a day or two later, after the results of microscopy and staining.

(c)   Depigmentation and lipodystrophy are not uncommon, even after a single injection.

(d)   Beware! It may be a parotid lesion and the close proximity of the branches of the facial nerve does not make it 'easy'.

(e)   Thenar wasting warrants early decompression to prevent progression. I would make an urgent referral and inject to relieve the symptoms while the patient is awaiting the appointment.

Q11(e) Refer immediately to the plastic surgeons, preferably by phoning directly. If definitive treatment is done within 3 to 4 weeks of excision, it does not affect prognosis.

Q13(b) A verruca is not a corn! How will you distinguish a verruca from a corn?

Q14(c) 3:1 with at least 2 mm clearance, especially in doubtful lesions.

Q15(d) Thenar motor branch of the median nerve.

Q17(a) HBV is highly infectious. 0.00004 ml of blood can transfer infections in humans. A larger volume is needed to transmit HIV, at least 0.1 ml (BMA. *A Code of Practice for the Safe Use and Disposal of Sharps*. London, BMA; 1993).

Q18(a) –20°C

(b) CO_2 snow = –79°C

(c)   –20°C

(d)   –75°C

Q20(d) 15 compressions for two inflations.

(e)   Best done just prior to the surgery. If done too early, the trauma of shaving can potentially cause the skin organisms to multiply.

Index